Contents

Foreword   vii

Acknowledgments   ix

Executive summary   xi

1   Introduction   1

   1.1 Aims of the review   3

2   Understanding breastfeeding   4

   2.1 The context of breastfeeding   6

   2.2 Physiology and psychological processes   6
      Supply and demand   6
      Let down   7
      Physiological ability to produce milk 8
      Social and psychological factors   8

   2.3 The development of the present 'bottle feeding' culture   9
      Key Practice Area A: A positive informed attitude to breastfeeding   11

3   Methods of the review   12

   3.1 Inclusion/exclusion criteria   12

   3.2 Search strategy   12

   3.3 Preparation of material   12

4   Results of the review   15

   4.1 Interventions intended to support breastfeeding, or which may   15
      interfere with breastfeeding
      Antenatal care   15
      Antenatal expression of colostrum   16
      Nipple preparation   17
      Treatment for inverted and non-protractile nipples   19
      Care after birth – routines which may prevent or cause clinical   21
        problems

Timing of the first feed 22
Prevention of sore nipples 26
Key Practice Area B: Professional assistance with positioning 30
and attachment
Key Practice Area C: Pain-free, effective feeding 31
Frequency and duration of breastfeeding 33
'Supplementing' the baby 36
Key Practice Area D: Professional assistance with flexible patterns 37
of feeding
Methods of giving additional fluids 44
Use of pacifiers (dummies) with breastfed babies 45
Key Practice Area E: No routine use of bottle, teats, dummies and 48
nipple shields
Giving discharge packs of formula 49

5 Common breastfeeding problems **52**

5.1 **Sore nipples and breasts** 52
Sore nipples 52
Nipple shields 53
Breast shells 53
Dressings (and other applications) 53
Infection 54
Sore breasts 54

5.2 **Problems with milk flow** 56
Breast engorgement 56
Mastitis 58

5.3 **Problems with milk supply** 62
Causes of 'insufficient milk' 64
Prevention of 'insufficient milk' 66
Treatment of 'insufficient milk' 67

6 Baby-related problems **73**

6.1 **Hypoglycaemia** 73
Routine management of asymptomatic babies 73
Management of the baby who doesn't wake to feed 74
'Symptomatic' hypoglycaemia 74
Babies at risk of hypoglycaemia 75
Routine management 75
Clinically relevant levels 75
Mechanism of testing 75

6.2 **Jaundice** 77

6.3 **Crying and 'colic'** 79

6.4 Down's syndrome   81

6.5 Cleft lip and palate   82

6.6 Tongue tie (ankyloglossia)   84
     Key Practice Area F: Practising evidence-based care in maternity units   86

6.7 Summary of baby problems   87

7 General discussion and future research priorities   88

8 Summary of recommendations for future research   91
     Urgent research areas   91
     Important research areas   92
     Costs associated with infant feeding and its problems   93

9 References   95

Appendices   115
     I. Details of search strategy   117
     II. Tables   121

Foreword

Very rarely does successful and painless breastfeeding happen without any help. It requires the patience and dedication of both health professionals and the mothers themselves. And, of course, the support of the mother's family. *Enabling Women to Breastfeed* provides an invaluable source of advice for health professionals to draw on and which should help to ensure that each baby has the opportunity to start its life with natural advantages.

One of the underpinning themes of this Government's health policies is the provision of accurate and consistent information to enable people themselves to make healthy lifestyle choices. *Enabling Women to Breastfeed* provides health professionals with guidance, based on a structured literature review, to ensure that mothers get consistent advice on how to tackle some of the problems they may encounter when trying to breastfeed their babies.

I know that this source of information will make a difference to today's mothers who want to breastfeed and for the generations of mothers to come.

Sarah Mullally
CHIEF NURSING OFFICER/DIRECTOR OF NURSING

Acknowledgements

We are very grateful for the input and comments of colleagues. Dr Jim Akre, Chloe Fisher, Sandra Lang, Maureen Minchin, Dr Felicity Savage-King, Dr Mary Smale, and Dr Tony Williams acted as critical readers. Their suggestions were very valuable and enhanced the quality of the review. Responsibility for any errors, however, remains ours.

In addition to acting as a critical reviewer, Dr Mary Smale assisted with additional discussion and writing. Further thanks are due to Dr Tony Williams for permitting us to read and cite his review of Hypoglycaemia. We are also grateful for the feedback received from Cynthia Rickitt and members of the National Network of Breastfeeding Coordinators on the evidence-based recommendations for practice.

Saira Dunnakey helped to design the search strategy, and gave valuable teaching on systematic searching. Liz Floyd gave very helpful input to preparing the original report, including editing the tables. We are also enormously grateful to the following people for their valuable input during the earlier stages of preparation of this document: John Berry, who cheerfully and industriously tracked down the literature we needed, Felicia McCormick who assisted with initial reviewing of papers, Trish Walker who provided administrative support to the project, and to Julie Batchelor for final presentation of the original draft.

The Department of Health funded Helen Ross McGill's work on this project.

Executive Summary

The aims of this structured literature review were to identify and review research studies in which interventions that enable women to continue to breastfeed or which interfere with the continuation of breastfeeding have been examined. On the basis of this information, the aim was both to produce a set of practice recommendations which are evidence-based and to identify questions for future research.

A total of 121 research studies were identified as appropriate for review, including those published up to and including December 1997. Details of these papers are given in individual tables appended to the text. Topics covered include antenatal preparation, routine care after birth, common breastfeeding problems and baby-related feeding problems.

Research

The volume of research covered by this review might give the erroneous impression that there is sufficient firm evidence available to inform practice. In fact, the most striking finding is the paucity of good, well-designed research to inform an area of health care which has profound short and long term effects on such large numbers of people. These gaps are especially apparent in relation to the leading causes of breastfeeding discontinuation; 'insufficient milk', and sore nipples and breasts. Factors underlying the scarcity of relevant, high quality research include the following: studies have not addressed some of the key practical issues in the field; many studies are too small to be useful, or are methodologically flawed; studies examining biomedical questions seldom consider the fundamental contribution of support, information and advice, the effects of women's views and feelings, and the social and cultural context of breastfeeding; and most studies reviewed took place in a culture when breastfeeding practices and routines were such that a large proportion of problems were a result of mismanagement. As a result, some very simple questions have not been addressed.

Future research in this field would benefit from dividing the issues into two major areas: issues which are common and widespread, affecting large numbers of women and babies, such as engorgement, 'insufficient milk', sore nipples and crying babies; and issues which are much less common, but result in distress and discontinuation of breastfeeding. The three specific research areas which need to be most urgently addressed are:

- the widespread problem of 'milk insufficiency' needs a programme of work to address the interrelated physical, psychological, social and cultural problems
- why is it difficult to change practice in areas where research has demonstrated potential dramatic improvements for mothers and babies, and what would help to support such changes?
- pain-free, effective feeding is fundamental to successful breastfeeding and research is urgently needed to examine training programmes for caregivers to educate them in this essential skill.

In addition, an analysis of the costs associated with infant feeding and its problems would demonstrate the scale of the demands on the health service which result from the present situation. This would require a full risk-assessment analysis of the various health outcomes associated with different methods of infant feeding.

Practice

Recommendations for professional practice are made based on the evidence reviewed. The general implications of these practice recommendations are that more staff time and training are needed in order to support those women effectively who start to breastfeed.

A coordinated approach to practice and research, involving the full range of professionals who work with mothers and babies, and the agencies involved in funding research in this field, is needed to address this urgent problem. Such an approach has succeeded in other countries.

1 Introduction

The health gains from prolonged, exclusive breastfeeding are universally acknowledged. The challenge for healthcare professionals and other caregivers is how to enable women who start to breastfeed to continue to do so, and thereby to benefit from the health outcomes.

In a traditional rural setting in the developing world, cultural practices, such as the early introduction of weaning foods, can be the sole hindrance to achieving exclusive breastfeeding, as it is usually prolonged by Western standards. In contrast, it is unfortunately the case that in an urban industrialised setting, professional practices have often been the main barrier to the successful establishment of breastfeeding. What factors are important, therefore, in enabling women to breastfeed successfully, and what practices have been shown either to help or to hinder the establishment of breastfeeding? The answers to such questions are important for women, for their babies, for caregivers, and for the healthcare system – purchasers and policy-makers alike.

Successive quinquennial surveys in the United Kingdom have shown that the incidence and prevalence of breastfeeding have remained largely static since 1980. The most recent national figures available, from the survey carried out in 1995 (Foster et al 1997) showed that 66% of women started to breastfeed. By six weeks after birth only 42% of women were still breastfeeding and many of these were also giving additional feeds of formula. This sharp decline in the maintenance of breastfeeding has shown no improvement since 1980 (Martin & Monk 1982, Martin & White 1988, White et al 1992, Foster et al 1997). This is a consequence of the fact that many women are encountering problems and stopping before they wish to (Foster et al 1997), in association with which they exhibit low emotional wellbeing (Green et al 1998). Women and their babies are deprived of the health benefits from prolonged breastfeeding and the health service incurs increased costs both from the resource use in caring for women encountering feeding problems and the economic burden from treating infections and other medical conditions arising from artificial feeding.

In contrast to the United Kingdom, the rates of breastfeeding have increased over the last decade in several European countries (most notably Scandinavia) and other industrialised nations (such as Canada, Australia, New Zealand), in some cases from very low levels; in Norway 80% of women are still breastfeeding three months after birth (Rosenberg, 1989). This demonstrates that it is possible to reverse the situation that applies in the UK, even in cultures where bottle feeding has been the norm (Helsing & Kjäernes 1985, Baumslag and Michels 1995).

Many authors have attempted to address the problem since the decline in breastfeeding started some 40 years ago and a plethora of books exists together with leaflets for mothers and health professionals on breastfeeding. The past two decades have seen dramatic changes in the advice given about how to breastfeed, shifting from a reliance on tradition and received wisdom, to placing greater weight on evidence (Inch and Renfrew 1989). Nonetheless, it remains difficult for caregivers to be confident that they are giving women appropriate evidence-based advice, which will ensure problem-free breastfeeding, and for women to be confident that they have been given the soundest possible advice, which will guarantee them success if put into practice.

Providing support, information and consistent advice for women has been shown to be effective in helping women to continue to breastfeed (Sikorski and Renfrew 1999). Such care is not always available, however, and women often experience inconsistent advice about breastfeeding practice or irreconcilable advice on how to resolve specific problems. This view was supported by the Audit Commission report (Garcia et al 1998) which suggested that a proportion of mothers are not receiving active support and encouragement with breastfeeding postnatally (18% in hospital, 10% at home), or enough practical help (16% in hospital, 13% at home), and still receive inconsistent advice (24% in hospital, 14% at home) (table 21 in Garcia et al 1998).

We should not be surprised when such irreconcilable advice results in confusion and the discontinuation of breastfeeding. For example, on the one hand, women are likely to be advised to breastfeed exclusively and to avoid giving their babies any supplementary milk, while on the other, to offer 'top-ups' of formula if their babies cannot be settled by breastfeeding alone. Women may be encouraged by some health professionals to use creams and ointments antenatally to prepare their nipples and breasts for breastfeeding, but be told by others to avoid any such preparations altogether. Mothers may be encouraged to feed their baby immediately after birth, to wait until they have been sutured, or their baby is clean, or even until they get back to the postnatal ward, but not when their baby is ready – the most opportune moment. They may be told to feed from one breast only at each feed, or to make sure that they use both breasts equally. Advice which is either inconsistent or is given without any rationale, does not offer women any basis by which they can reach informed choices

In order to resolve such inconsistencies, it is important to examine critically what evidence exists and what it has to tell us. This structured review, commissioned by the Department of Health, aims to examine evidence relating to interventions which support or inhibit breastfeeding. Research studies were reviewed without setting restrictions on their methodology.

Much of the evidence described in this paper is not new, some of it being several decades old. By examining critically all the studies together in one review, our intention was both to demonstrate areas where evidence is secure enough to produce recommendations for practice and to identify where new research is needed.

1.1 Aims of the review

The aims of this review were:

1. To identify and review research studies in which factors that enable women to continue to breastfeed or which interfere with the continuation of breastfeeding have been examined.

2. On the basis of this information:
   i.   to highlight implications for practice,
   ii   to identify questions for future research.

The specific factors to be identified and included were:
- Interventions (including practices, drugs, and devices) intended to promote or sustain breastfeeding, or which may interfere with it. This includes care which may prevent clinical problems, or which may be the cause of them.
- Routine treatments for common problems of breastfeeding such as engorgement, sore nipples, mastitis and 'insufficient milk'.
- Support for women who wish to breastfeed infants with potential feeding difficulties, such as cleft lip and palate and infants with Downs syndrome.

Several topics and issues were regarded as falling outside the scope of this review, such as the care of sick and premature babies and feeding twins or higher-order multiple births.

The cultural context of breastfeeding can have a profound effect on the implementation of effective care and on whether ineffective and harmful practices are prevented. Similarly, the attitudes of women themselves, of their caregivers and families, and the quality of support women do, or do not, receive when they breastfeed all exert an influence on the outcome of breastfeeding. These topics were regarded as outside the remit of this review, but some of the relevant literature has been drawn on in the discussion and recommendations. We hope this will assist readers of this report to set the interventions we discuss in context.

Several general issues have been summarised in the introductory section on 'Understanding Breastfeeding', including (i) the health outcomes associated with breastfeeding, (ii) the physiological mechanisms involved in lactation, and (iii) reasons for the discontinuation of breastfeeding. These topics were included as they were considered fundamental to an understanding of the context of the research studies reviewed. They are also needed to inform the analysis of the material and to assist in the discussion of the strengths and deficiencies of existing research.

2 Understanding breastfeeding

Human breastmilk is a unique and valuable resource. It provides babies with a source of nutrition that changes in synchrony with each baby's growing needs. Breastfeeding is the natural method for providing breastmilk. It protects babies from common childhood infections (Cunningham et al 1992 for review, Wright et al 1989, Howie et al 1990, Duncan et al 1993) by mechanisms which are interactive, adaptive and long-lasting, and which extend into childhood (Wilson et al 1998). Breastfeeding also protects the baby from developing a range of diseases in later life (Saarinen & Kajosaari 1995), protection which is particularly important where there is an underlying predisposition to disease, for example, an established familial risk (Lucas et al 1990). Breastfeeding also offers the natural circumstances for the development of close, affectionate ties between the mother and her child. In addition to this, breastfeeding can act as an effective and safe means of birth spacing (Gray et al 1990), if certain guidelines are adhered to (Kennedy et al 1989), whilst also appearing to protect women against certain forms of cancer (pre-menopausal breast cancer – UKNCCSG 1993, epithelial ovarian cancer – Rosenblatt & Thomas 1993). There is widespread acceptance of the evidence for the health benefits arising from prolonged exclusive breastfeeding and recognition of the far-reaching public health benefits (Standing Committee on Nutrition of the British Paediatric Association 1994, Ministry of Agriculture, Fisheries and Food 1994, Faculty of Public Health Medicine 1995, Department of Health 1995).

Replacing breastfeeding is impossible; while it is possible to feed babies with artificial substitutes, many of the attributes of breastfeeding are lost as a result. In addition to the loss of the health benefits described, potential adverse side effects of feeding artificial substitutes include contamination (Miller & Chopra 1984) inaccurate preparation of feeds resulting in over- or under-concentration of nutrients (Taitz & Byers 1972, Smith 1974, Lucas et al 1992), and an increased use of resources (Walker 1993).

In spite of the proven advantages of breastfeeding, as many as 35% of women in the UK do not start to breastfeed their babies. Figures for the incidence and prevalence of breastfeeding, available from the most recent national survey conducted in 1995 (Foster et al 1997), indicate that there has been no substantive change since the second survey in 1980. Between 1990 and 1995 there was an apparent increase (close to 4%) in both the initiation rate for breastfeeding and its prevalence at 6 weeks. However, once corrected for the age structure of the population the trend shows that the proportion of women starting to breastfeed has remained static at 62%[1] and the same is likely to be true of the six week rate (Martin and Monk 1982, Martin and White 1988, White et al 1992, Foster et al 1997). So although the majority of new mothers in the UK choose to breastfeed their newborn baby, only a minority (26%) reach the minimum age at which the introduction of complementary foods is recommended to be considered (4–6 months, WHO/UNICEF 1980, WHO 1995).

The reasons for the low initiation rate may include the woman's cultural background and her expectations, a personal or socially-imposed distaste for breastfeeding (McIntosh 1985), difficult previous experiences, or her intention to return to work (Martin and White 1988, Foster et al 1997). For those women who start, it remains the case that many encounter problems and stop before they wish to, with as few as 2.6% of women who stop breastfeeding under four months stating that they had breastfed 'for long enough' or 'for as long as they had intended' (White et al 1992). Women who encounter difficulties, who may stop as a result, experience feelings of guilt and distress (Houston 1984).

Overall, these figures represent a chronic failure by the healthcare system to provide women with the help and support they need to implement the widespread recommendation that exclusive breastfeeding till 4–6 months is ideal. The steep decline in breastfeeding rate should be a particular cause of concern as it means that babies are deprived of the health benefits of breastfeeding and exposed to the hazards of artificial milk substitutes. Women experience distress and the health services have additional demands imposed. **A good analysis of the costs associated with infant feeding would help to establish the costs of this situation to the National Health Service; these costs are likely to be very high.**

For example, approximately 700,000 women give birth annually in England and Wales. By four months after birth, only 230,000 women will still be breastfeeding. The 300,000 women, and babies, who stopped breastfeeding in that time have experienced a range of problems related to both themselves and their babies for which they will have consulted midwives, health visitors, GPs and paediatricians. The health services will also have increased demands in the long term, related to health problems such as gastro-intestinal illness, respiratory infection and otitis media for babies who were not breastfed (Howie et al 1990, Duncan et al 1993). The differential demands placed on health services persist throughout adolescence, as shown by a follow-up study of Scottish children experiencing increased respiratory morbidity at seven years of age from not being exclusively breastfed (Wilson et al 1998). In preventative health terms the figures represent a huge lost potential; for the ability of breastfeeding to make a genuine contribution to the health of our nation, they verge on a national disaster.

---

[1] Standardised for mother's age and age at which she finished full-time education (Foster et al. 1997).

The rapid discontinuation is not inevitable. The leading causes of discontinuation given by women are insufficient milk supply, painful breasts or nipples, the baby would not suck or rejected the breast, and mothers feeling that breastfeeding took too long or was tiring (White et al 1992, Foster et al, 1997). The evidence summarised in this paper suggests that for many women these problems can be prevented, while those experiencing such problems can continue to breastfeed successfully, given accurate advice and good support.

2.1 The context of breastfeeding

Any analysis of breastfeeding problems and the factors which may influence them must be considered within the context of an understanding of the physiological processes underlying breastfeeding and of the social and psychological influences which affect women, their families, health professionals, and indeed everyone in the wider social context. It is not possible to disentangle the effects of specific practices and interventions from the context in which they are provided. For example, a number of interventions were carried out in the 1940s and 1950s by Waller and his colleagues in the British Hospital for Mothers and Babies in London, including antenatal expression of colostrum and preparation of inverted nipples. Some of these practices appeared to have been successful. The context of this care, however, was a very supportive environment, in which women were taught about breastfeeding and supported by experienced midwifery and medical staff. Would such practices have worked without the support and education? It would only be possible to know that if further research was carried out in a non-supportive culture. It is likely, however, that the knowledge of the health professionals involved, their beliefs in the value and feasibility of breastfeeding and the skilled support they provided, all influenced the outcome.

The following sections will summarise briefly the physiological processes and the context of breastfeeding in the UK today, as a framework for the interpretation of the results of this review.

2.2 Physiological and psychological processes

A number of fundamental physiological processes underlie the successful production of milk and its transfer to the baby. These processes are well described by Akre 1989, Hamosh and Goldman 1986, and Woolridge 1995 and will be summarised here very briefly.

Supply and demand

Hormonal control of milk synthesis

Milk production is controlled primarily by three factors. In the early days and weeks, prolactin is released in response to feeding and has a role in establishing the broad limits to milk output. Once peak milk output is achieved at around five weeks, control of milk supply seems to be regulated mostly by autocrine control and the baby's appetite.

Autocrine control   Milk is synthesised by the secretory cells in the alveoli. A milk fraction produced by these secretory cells acts locally to inhibit output of those cells (Peaker & Wilde, 1987, 1995, Wilde et al 1995). As milk builds up in the breast between feeds, a factor in the milk (termed the Feedback Inhibitor of Lactation – FIL) works to slow milk synthesis by exerting negative feedback. If milk is not removed effectively and regularly milk production will be inhibited.

Appetite control   Increasingly it is becoming recognised that the baby, if given the opportunity, exerts the ultimate control over milk supply. Several studies (Fomon et al 1975, Woolridge et al 1980, Dewey and Lonnerdal 1986, Dewey et al 1991) have demonstrated the existence of an appetite control mechanism, by which the baby regulates either fat or calorie intake to achieve a steady consumption over time. The message is that if culturally-imposed limitations on feeding exist, such as restrictions on the frequency or duration of feeds, the baby will not be able to regulate his or her intake appropriately. Such limitations prevent the baby from securing his or her nutritional needs and a range of problems may result, including slow weight gain, crying, or symptoms of colic.

In summary, therefore, the amount of milk removed by the baby is related to the amount of milk subsequently synthesized by the mother and adequate milk synthesis depends on effective and frequent removal of milk from the breast (Daly et al 1992, Daly et al 1993). This key physiological principle underlies many of the practices described in this paper, as any factor which interferes with effective milk removal will interfere with the mother's subsequent ability to synthesize more milk for her baby. In the absence of factors which might disrupt the normal physiological regulation of milk supply, the baby's appetite will naturally control the amount of milk produced, thus balancing demand and supply. If the system is in balance the mother should not experience excessive fullness or shortage of milk for her baby and she should also be able to breastfeed twins or triplets if necessary. If the system is not in balance, problems may result which can include engorgement, a low milk supply, slow weight gain or weight loss in the baby, and a hungry, crying baby.

Let-down

Milk synthesised in the breast is stored in the alveoli and then actively released by the action of the hormone oxytocin. Oxytocin is released by the action of the baby feeding, but is also responsive to psychological factors such as the mother hearing her baby cry, or knowing that her baby wants to feed (McNeilly 1977). The release of oxytocin can be inhibited by psychological factors such as stress, although the only empirical research identified on the relationship between stress and oxytocin inhibition was a study using the sudden severe stressors of electric shock and plunging the mother's feet into a bucket of ice (Newton and Newton 1948). Questions remain over whether or not less severe stress inhibits oxytocin in the same way and for how long any such inhibition lasts.

Physiological ability to produce milk

The number of women who are incapable of producing enough milk to feed their babies is not known accurately, but there is good evidence that in the right circumstances almost all women are capable of producing an adequate milk supply. In societies in which breastfeeding is regarded as a natural physiological function, where it is the only way to nourish an infant, where it is highly valued, strongly encouraged and supported by society in general and families in particular, lactation failure is much less common, and partial breastfeeding at least commonly continues into the second year or beyond (Akre 1989). The rapid discontinuation of breastfeeding in the first few weeks after the birth of the baby, therefore, is not the result of a widespread biological inability to produce enough milk, but is more likely to be the result of cultural factors and practices.

Social and psychological factors

These issues have been well summarised in a number of publications, including Allen and Pelto 1986, Minchin 1998, Palmer 1993, Lawrence 1994 and Riordan and Auerbach 1993. A general overview only will be given here.

Breastfeeding is far from being simply a physiological process. It also involves a dynamic psychological relationship between mother and child, affecting the behaviour and emotions of both mother and baby. It takes place within the social and emotional context of the family, and other family members' responses to it. It also takes place in the wider social context, where the reactions and views of the extended family, neighbours, friends, strangers encountered in public places and even views expressed in the media may have an influence. In a culture where breastfeeding is the norm, these strong community influences on breastfeeding are likely to have a positive and reinforcing effect. In a culture where bottle feeding is the norm, and where confidence in women's ability to breastfeed is low, a strong negative effect is likely to result. In such a social context, information about practices which will enhance breastfeeding will have a limited impact.

Bottles, teats, sterilisation and infant formula have developed sufficiently in this century to enable mothers to use them with comparative ease, although there are a number of practical problems associated with bottle feeding such as the need for cleanliness, access to safe water and accurate preparation of feeds which may provide challenges. Many women find that bottle feeding is acceptable in a public setting in a way in which breastfeeding is not. Parents rarely have the opportunity to see breastfeeding before their own baby is born. Dolls with bottles or dummies, symbols on changing rooms, all demonstrate the 'normality' of the process of bottle-feeding and, by implication, the 'abnormality' of breastfeeding. Despite some legislation about advertising to parents, the names of formula manufacturers are frequently visible to women on educational pamphlets and posters about pregnancy and childcare, and the pens, calendars and diaries used by health professionals.

Health professionals, of course, are not immune to the influences of the culture in which they live and work. A number of studies have indicated a range of views among health professionals about the benefits of breastfeeding, and whether women should be strongly recommended to breastfeed (for example, Freed et al 1995). As a result, health professionals are likely to vary in the quality of advice they give, in the overt or covert messages they give to women about the importance of continuing, and in the confidence they have that the woman can succeed in the face of problems. They are also likely to vary in the use they make of evidence derived from research, especially if it conflicts with personal or long-held beliefs. **The beliefs and attitudes of health professionals need urgent investigation, if the information derived from research and research reviews is to filter through to professional practice.**

One of the contributory factors in the development of both inaccurate, conflicting information and ambivalent attitudes among caregivers and the public may have been the previous lack of strong, convincing evidence about the health outcomes of infant feeding in industrialised countries and of the effects of interventions such as additional bottles or timing of feeds, on which to base knowledge and advice. This may be partly a result of methodological flaws in much of the existing research (Bauchner et al 1986, Cunningham 1988, Auerbach et al 1991) and the fact that much research in breastfeeding has been conducted in a limited biomedical context, in which social and psychological influences have not been considered. As a result, many crucial questions have not been asked.

2.3 The development of the present 'bottle feeding' culture

In the early decades of this century, as alternative baby foods started to become widely available, there was an effort in professional and lay publications to render breastfeeding 'scientific and exact'. There were a range of influences on this process, which have been well summarised by other writers (for example, Hardyment 1983 and Minchin 1998). A pervasive view, influencing both breastfeeding mothers and health professionals alike, was that the same degree of control and regulation which had been developed for the artificially-fed baby should now be imposed on the breastfed baby (Beekman, 1977). This also presupposed that the breastfeeding mother 'knew', and could be confident, that her baby was receiving a known, predictable and consistent amount. When her baby failed to comply with such time-regulated targets, the only assumption could be that she was failing to supply a reliable and adequate amount – so giving rise to the cultural myth of 'insufficient milk supply'. All these issues revealed a fundamental misunderstanding of the process by which the infant regulates milk supply by expressing his/her 'demand' for milk (by appetite-control); this erroneous view can still pervade current breastfeeding management.

Much of the widespread early discontinuation of breastfeeding that has occurred over the subsequent decades may be attributable to iatrogenic practices such as limiting spontaneous contact between the mother and her baby, the timing of feeds, test-weighing, and the giving of supplementary bottles of formula to breastfeeding babies. Decades of women learned either to use bottles as a part of breastfeeding or to turn to them when they 'failed' with breastfeeding.

These changes were, of course, set in a wider social context. For example, the interest in attempting to condition the baby's appetite by limiting the time mother and baby spent together has been examined as a part of a much wider attempt to industrialise society and to 'protect' mothers from their babies who might develop into monsters without discipline unless controlled (Hardyment 1983). The increasing need for women to work outside the home during both World Wars and the availability of 'National Dried Milk' have been seen as important influences on the development of artificial feeding (Royal College of Midwives, 1991).

A widespread lack of confidence in breastfeeding which resulted from these changes remains endemic throughout our culture, both collectively and individually. This lack of confidence is demonstrated by women in pregnancy who, when asked how they will feed, often reply that they will 'try' to breastfeed; it is also demonstrated by their families, peers and caregivers alike, being the source of often harsh and ambivalent attitudes to breastfeeding. Such ambivalence towards the value and desirability of breastfeeding was shown, for example, in one study of the attitudes of schoolchildren in Liverpool, who saw breastfeeding as healthier and more natural than bottle feeding, but more embarrassing, while bottle feeding was seen as more convenient and fashionable (Gregg 1989). It is important, therefore, to consider interventions which may increase the confidence that women, their families and the wider public have in breastfeeding, a confidence in which caregivers can lead by example.

In our culture it would appear that, in the presence of restrictive practices and the prejudicial views of the population at large, women do not have a free choice to breastfeed successfully – that is, while they may have made a free choice to initiate breastfeeding they cannot exercise the same choice over whether they continue. They will need support from healthcare workers, partners, relatives and friends alike to enable them to do so. They will also benefit from sound advice and practically-based education, both before and after the birth of their child.

Society at large needs to be educated into the health gains accruing from successful breastfeeding, how to manage the process effectively, and how to generate confidence and security in the knowledge that breastfeeding is a natural process which has worked in the past, and will continue to work, so long as it is freed from prescriptive advice and limitations.

Although outside the scope of this review, there are examples of interventions which demonstrate that it is possible to counteract these strong cultural effects, for example by a programme of antenatal education (Valdes et al 1993, Pugin et al 1996), by providing postnatal support (Houston et al 1981, Jenner 1988), or by a number of socio-political measures (Baumslag and Michels 1995).

KEY PRACTICE AREA A

Professional Assistance:
A positive, informed attitude to breastfeeding

Healthcare professionals and other caregivers who have contact with breastfeeding mothers and their babies require the technical expertise, skill and sensitivity to empower women to breastfeed successfully, combined with a positive attitude towards breastfeeding. Being confident in the breastfeeding process itself and in the capability of the mother to develop her own competence is likely to foster the same positive feelings in the women in their care.

It would not seem appropriate for the first point of contact between an expectant mother, or one who has newly delivered, to be with someone who has entrenched views or adverse attitudes towards breast-feeding. In view of the broad and long-lasting health benefits to both the mother and her infant from breastfeeding, the public health priority is to promote breastfeeding unequivocally within the healthcare system. Should a healthcare professional have any ambivalent or adverse personal views, based on their own experience, these should not be allowed to enter into, or to colour, their practice.

Nonetheless, it is important to remain aware that individual women may be personally ambivalent to, or have an antipathy towards breastfeeding – recognising that there may be some tangible basis for this in their past (such as sexual abuse as a child). It is important therefore for health professionals not to become over-zealous in promoting the public health message.

It may well be the case that all staff should be de-briefed on their own personal experience of, or attitudes towards infant feeding before they have routine contact with breastfeeding women. Facilities for counselling should be made available to both staff and women should they require access to such a facility.

No routine mechanisms exist for exploring staff experiences and attitudes, or those of women in their care. The routine provision of such facilities for either healthcare staff, or for women who wish to receive such assistance, should be seriously considered.

3 Methods of the review

The study was a structured literature review, which followed some of the conventions of a systematic review. Funding did not allow time for a full systematic analysis, however, and there may well be areas of literature which have not been adequately covered.

3.1 Inclusion/exclusion criteria

Only the English language literature was searched. The searches included studies from several decades; the majority of the studies, however, are from the past twenty years. Studies have been included regardless of the research method used.

3.2 Search strategy

The search strategy was developed with the support of Saira Dunnakey from the NHS Centre for Reviews and Dissemination, University of York. Both electronic and hand searches were carried out up to December 1997. Full details are given in Appendix I.

3.3 Preparation of material

All papers were read by the research midwife (HRM) and the researcher (MJR). A structured format was prepared to summarise each paper identified, and HRM prepared a summary table for each paper in consultation with MJR. Tables were also reviewed by the critical readers; final editing was checked by another researcher, Liz Floyd.

Studies were summarised in individual tables using the following headings:
    Title
    Research method
    Full citation
    Intervention assessed
        (controlled trials and other experimental studies only)

Details of methods used (descriptive studies only)
Entry criteria
Number of women and/or babies studied
Outcomes measured
Results

Resources did not allow systematic assessment of the methodological quality of each paper. Readers can assess the quality of the paper for themselves by reading the summary of the methods used in each Table. In addition, methodological quality is described in the text when this is relevant.

Papers identified One hundred and twenty one research studies were identified, published between 1945 and 1997. The great majority of these papers were reports of experimental studies. Papers included in the review were categorised according to the topic of the study, and the research method used. In summary, papers covered the following topics:

Topic	Number of papers	%
1. Antenatal care	10	8
2. Routine care in the initiation of breastfeeding	49	39
3. Common breastfeeding problems	56	44
4. Baby-related problems	12	9
TOTAL	**127***	**100**

The following research methods were used in the papers identified:

Research method used	Number of papers	%
1. Randomised controlled trials	57	46
2. Non-randomised prospective studies	42	34
3. Retrospective cohort studies/case-control studies/before–after studies	5	4
4. Surveys/literature reviews/descriptive or observational studies	13	10
5. Case studies	8	6
TOTAL	**125***	**100**

*These totals exceed 121 as some papers covered more than one topic, and some papers reported more than one study, sometimes using two or more research methods.

A total of 121 tables have therefore been prepared, summarising the studies identified; these are presented in full in Appendix II. Each table is numbered, and studies are identified in the text by this number in square brackets [ ], as well as by the names of the authors and date of publication. Information given in the text about each paper is brief; the reader may wish to examine the individual tables if full details are required.

Where necessary, appropriate background information is summarised in the text to set the interventions discussed in context.

On the basis of this evidence, recommendations for practice, and for further research, are given.

4 Results of the review

The results of the systematic search and analysis of the papers are presented in the following sections:

- Interventions intended to support breastfeeding, or which may interfere with breastfeeding. These include care which may prevent or cause clinical problems
- Treatment of common clinical problems
- Support for women who wish to breastfeed infants with potential feeding difficulties

Throughout this review, following presentation and discussion of the studies conducted in relation to each practice, we have produced a set of evidence-based *Practice Implications* for that topic to provide guidance for health professionals beside which they can evaluate their own current practice, and the policy under which they operate, in order to determine whether it is both up-to-date and evidence-based. These guidelines have been reviewed extensively by expert practitioners across the UK.

Some key issues arise so repeatedly that we feel they deserve to be recognised as core practices. We have, therefore, produced a small set of *Key Practice Areas*, with explanatory notes on how to interpret them; in certain instances such guidelines may not be based solely on evidence, although they are firmly grounded in best professional practice. These include:

Professional assistance with:

- a positive informed attitude to breastfeeding
- positioning and attachment
- pain-free, effective feeding
- flexible patterns of feeding
- no routine use of bottles, teats, dummies & nipple shields
- practising evidence-based care in maternity units

4.1 Interventions intended to support breastfeeding, or which may interfere with breastfeeding

Antenatal care

A range of practices have been recommended to pregnant women over the years, with the aim of increasing the duration of breastfeeding. Two main areas of care have been examined in research studies: antenatal expression of colostrum, and nipple preparation.

Antenatal expression of colostrum

Four studies on the routine expression of colostrum by women in pregnancy were identified (Waller 1946 [1], Blaikeley et al 1953 [2], Ingelmann-Sundberg 1958 [3], Brown and Hurlock 1975 [4]), three of which were carried out several decades ago. Details of the practice are not always given, but women appear to have been asked to express colostrum daily in the last trimester of pregnancy. The practice was first recommended by Waller (1946) to prepare women to express after birth to help relieve engorgement. In three of the studies (Waller 1946, Blaikeley et al 1953 and Ingelmann-Sundberg 1958) expression was preceded by breast massage.

Three of these studies were controlled trials (Waller 1946, Blaikeley et al 1953, Brown and Hurlock 1975), although in two (Waller 1946 and Blaikeley et al 1953) women were allocated alternately, rather than at random. The fourth study was a non-randomised cohort comparison (Ingleman-Sundberg et al 1958). Brown and Hurlock (1975) do not present any numerical results. The regimens differ, and expression was continued after birth in three of the four studies.

There is some suggestion from the results of these studies [Tables 1–4] that the antenatal expression of colostrum may result in an increase in the duration of breastfeeding and a decrease in the incidence of engorgement and sore nipples.

Discussion   It is perhaps surprising that the encouraging results of these studies have not resulted in further research. The results may be explained by other factors, however; for example, women in one study (Blaikeley et al 1953) also received other forms of care (for example, 'general advice on breastfeeding, advice on suitable brassieres, attention to nipples and treatment of them with glass shells where necessary'), and it is likely that women in both groups received additional attention from midwives and obstetricians after birth. There was a high rate of engorgement in both Waller's and Blaikeley's studies; these studies took place at a time when feeding times and duration were limited. It could be that antenatal expression combined with postnatal expression is an effective treatment for engorgement, but that prevention of engorgement by flexible feeding patterns is the best solution to that problem.

PRACTICE IMPLICATIONS:

• There is insufficient evidence of a specific benefit from antenatal expression of colostrum so the practice should not be encouraged. There is, however, no reason to advise against it should a woman wish to carry it out as a matter of personal choice.

Further research A well-designed randomised controlled trial of antenatal expression of colostrum, conducted in the setting of a modern hospital implementing up-to-date practices, would address the problems raised above concerning method and interpretation. Women are still routinely advised to wear a 'good supporting bra' both throughout pregnancy and lactation. To our knowledge this has not been evaluated by a controlled trial, although many women will elect to do this for reasons of comfort and personal choice.

Nipple preparation

Routine preparation of the nipples In the past, women were commonly encouraged to prepare their nipples in pregnancy, attempting to 'toughen', or condition them in order to prevent pain when the baby started to feed. Studies do not indicate that any such regime has been helpful. Hewat and Ellis (1987) [5] carried out a non-randomised prospective study in which 23 women were asked to express breastmilk onto one nipple and use hydrous lanolin on the other. Ninety-five percent of the women experienced nipple pain and there was no perceived difference between the two treatments.

Storr (1988) [6] asked 25 women to carry out 'nipple rolling' for 30 seconds twice a day and to rub the nipple lightly with a towel. Women acted as their own controls: they were asked to prepare one breast only. The results showed less tenderness with the prepared nipple; the study was very small, however, and several methodological problems of the study were raised by the author herself.

Brown and Hurlock (1975) [4] compared nipple rolling, the application of Massé cream and the expression of colostrum. Again, women acted as their own controls; the nipple to be conditioned was chosen by tossing a coin. No significant differences were found between the different treatments. Atkinson (1979) [7] and Fleming (1984) [8] both carried out small studies (22 and 17 women respectively) with women acting as their own controls by 'conditioning' one nipple and not the other. Women were asked to carry out a regime which included nipple rolling, gentle friction with a terry cloth towel and allowing the outer clothing to rub against the nipple. Although women reported less pain from the 'conditioned' nipple, no conclusions can be drawn as a result of the study design, the small numbers of women included, and flaws in the data analysis. Three other small and methodologically flawed studies (Clark 1985 [9], Whitley 1978 [10] and l'Esperance 1980 [11]) have also failed to show any effects of nipple conditioning.

Discussion There is no evidence to support the conditioning of nipples in pregnancy. Since cineradiographic and ultrasound studies have shown that the well-positioned nipple is protected from friction, and therefore from pain, by being drawn to the back of the baby's mouth (Ardran et al 1958, Smith et al 1985, Weber et al 1986), the emphasis has shifted away from 'toughening' or conditioning nipples, towards preventing the cause of trauma (Woolridge 1986b). Women, therefore, should not be encouraged to carry out such conditioning, which some may find painful or distasteful.

It is argued that expectant women should be encouraged to regard touching or handling their breasts as normal and, while antenatal expression may be a way of achieving this, the small number of studies conducted have shown no clear benefit. Nonetheless, should a woman wish to adopt a particular method as a matter of personal choice, or staff perceive that there may be some emotional benefit to her personally, then as long as she has been made aware that it is unlikely to be of any therapeutic benefit, on the basis of informed choice (and the probability that it is unlikely to cause harm), she should not be prevented from doing so. It should also be made clear to her that even if she were to believe this practice to have been of personal benefit to her, she should not encourage other women to adopt it.

PRACTICE IMPLICATIONS:

- As no method of antenatal nipple preparation has been shown to have a beneficial effect on the continuation of breastfeeding this practice should be abandoned. If an individual woman wishes to adopt any method as a matter of personal choice, she should be made aware of the lack of evidence for a therapeutic benefit. But, on the basis that it is unlikely to cause harm, she should not be discouraged from doing so.

Healthcare workers might consider the potential benefit of exploring an individual woman's attitudes towards her own breasts, and towards breastfeeding. If she expresses strong feelings against breastfeeding, or discomfort about handling her breasts, suggesting that she seeks specialised counselling support to address such issues may prove helpful (this is untested by research, as yet).

Further research   There is no indication that further research on routine nipple conditioning would be of benefit. Questions remain, however, about women who may be especially susceptible to developing sore nipples, including women with persistent dry or sensitive skin, or a history of dermatitis or eczema of the nipple and areola.

There is increasing concern for the number of women who have been sexually abused during their adolescence and who may, in consequence, have deeply entrenched feelings about their breasts and about them being handled. Healthcare staff should be aware of this possibility and be sensitive to such issues. If such a woman were identified it would be appropriate to offer her counselling, rather than either to ignore the issue or to advise her to feed her baby artificially. Methods for identification of women at risk and the efficacy of counselling in such situations is an important area for research.

Treatment for inverted and non-protractile nipples

In the past, women with inverted or non-protractile nipples were told that they may not be able to breastfeed, and women with either of these conditions may have a genuine worry that it will be more difficult for their baby to take the breast effectively. Hytten (1954) and Alexander et al (1992) have suggested that around 7–10% of women may have unilateral or bilateral inverted or non-protractile nipples. Treatments include breast shells (sometimes known as Woolwich shells), nipple-stretching exercises (sometimes known as Hoffman's exercises), surgery and use of a newly-developed device known as the 'Niplette'.

Two randomised trials have examined Hoffman's exercises and breast shells (Alexander et al 1992 [12], MAIN trial collaborative group 1994 [13]). A total of 559 women were recruited to these trials, which were run in the UK and Canada. The results of both trials showed no increase in the duration of breastfeeding in women who used either of the treatments, or indeed both in combination. Women reported a dislike of the treatments. The authors of the first study suggested that routine examination of the breasts in pregnancy be discontinued as a result (Alexander et al 1992). It was notable that 45% of women in the MAIN trial (1994) breastfed for at least six weeks, indicating that flat and inverted nipples are not a contraindication to breastfeeding.

One paper describes the use of surgery in improving the breastfeeding outcome for women with inverted nipples (Terrill and Stapelton 1991 [14]). Case studies of 5 pregnant women were described, who had surgical 'correction' of their inverted nipples, with or without division of the lactiferous ducts (no details are given about this procedure). Three women went on to breastfeed; two did not attempt breastfeeding on the advice of their surgeons. Two women who had had their lactiferous ducts divided did breastfeed, although both had difficulty. The numbers of women included in this study are too small to reach any conclusions, but there is some indication that division of the lactiferous ducts is not a total contraindication to breastfeeding.

The non-surgical correction of flat and inverted nipples, either ante-natally or between pregnancies, has been proposed by the 'suction method' (Gangal & Gangal 1978). Kesaree et al (1993 [15]) employed simple modification of a standard syringe to draw out inverted nipples prior to the baby attaching to the breast. In a case series of eight hospitalised babies, six proceeded to exclusive breastfeeding within 2–6 weeks, while a seventh, who was over six months of age, received solids in addition to being breastfed.

Use of the 'Niplette' device is described in one paper (McGeorge 1994 [16]). This device comprises a nipple mould (which comes in one standard size) to be placed over the nipple and areola complex; suction is then applied by withdrawing air using an 8ml syringe. Case histories of 14 pregnant women who went on to breastfeed were described. All are described as breastfeeding 'without difficulty'. Trauma to the nipple caused by the Niplette was described, attributed by the author of the paper to the women 'applying too much pressure' (McGeorge

1994). Although based on theoretical principles which have been tested in other areas of plastic surgery, the device has not been subjected to clinical evaluation.

Discussion   There is no evidence to support the use of any antenatal treatment for inverted or non-protractile nipples, or even to support antenatal breast examination to identify women with this condition. Breast shells and the Niplette device are readily available in major chain stores selling goods for mothers and babies, and women who are anxious about their nipples may purchase them 'just in case'. Breast shells have, however, been shown to be ineffective and the 'Niplette' device has not been adequately evaluated.

One encouraging finding from these studies is that a high proportion of women with inverted and non-protractile nipples in the trials did manage to breastfeed and women should be reassured that such a condition does not contraindicate breastfeeding. Women in these trials also described how distressing this condition can be and the lengths to which they were prepared to go to ensure they could breastfeed their babies.

It has been reported that gentle sucking stimuli to the inverted or flat nipple, for example by toddlers or sexual partners, may help to increase protractility. Evidence for this is lacking and it is a difficult and sensitive area to study. Women who are not averse to doing this may, however, find it helpful and it is unlikely to have adverse side effects.

PRACTICE IMPLICATIONS:

- All women should be reassured that it is possible to breastfeed successfully with inverted or non-protractile nipples.

- Given the lack of evidence for antenatal nipple preparation no specific practice can be recommended. There are also therefore no grounds for midwives to continue routine antenatal breast examination to identify conditions requiring treatment.

- Women who express concern about the shape of their nipples should be given extra support postnatally with positioning and attachment. They should also be offered assistance with breast expression to ensure both their milk supply and the baby's intake are adequate if attachment is especially difficult.

- Practices which may enhance the baby's ability to latch-on (e.g. use of a breast pump to draw the nipple out prior to feeding) may be attempted. Such practices are untested – it is unlikely that they cause harm if done gently and they may help.

- In contrast, professionals should exercise due caution against recommending methods which are as yet untested and which have the potential to cause harm.

- A woman who believes she was previously unsuccessful with breastfeeding because of inverted nipples, may elect for an as yet untested method (e.g. corrective surgery, 'Niplette'). If she does so she should be advised of possible adverse consequences, and to complete surgical treatment prior to a subsequent pregnancy.

Further research
- Use of the 'Niplette' device should be evaluated by a randomised controlled trial to examine its effectiveness, possible harmful side effects and the views of women who use it.
- Descriptive studies are needed to investigate the support and care needed by women who have inverted and non-protractile nipples in the early days and weeks after birth, to support them in the initiation and maintenance of breastfeeding and to explore ways of helping babies to take the breast effectively.
- In the light of the lack of evidence to support any antenatal treatments in pregnancy, a descriptive study of the views of women on the care they would like to receive in pregnancy to prepare them for breastfeeding is needed. Women may, for example, find it helpful to talk about breastfeeding, or to become familiar with handling their own breasts and nipples.

Care after birth –
routines which may prevent or cause clinical problems

A number of routine practices, not specifically related to breastfeeding, have been implicated over the years as interfering with the mother's ability to breast-feed her baby. These include separation of the mother from her baby after birth, gastric suctioning of the newborn, administration to the baby of prophylactic silver nitrate eye drops, and drugs given to the mother in labour. We have not reviewed these practices in detail here as research, reviewed by Inch and Garforth (1989), Bernard-Bonnin et al (1989), Perez-Escamilla et al (1992) and Vallenas & Savage (WHO 1998), indicated that the routine use of any of these practices was detrimental to breastfeeding and had no benefit as a routine form of care. It is therefore assumed that:
- mothers and babies will not be separated after birth, unless the mother requests it, or there is a problem that requires it. Every effort will be made to keep mother and baby in close proximity, even if the mother or her baby is unwell.
- no unnecessary routine practices will be carried out on the baby, especially if these have been shown to be detrimental to breastfeeding. These include gastric suctioning and prophylactic eye drops.
- care will be taken with administration of drugs to the mother in labour, to minimise the effects on her baby and subsequent effects on breastfeeding.

Timing of the first feed

Practices in the timing of the first breastfeed vary widely from culture to culture, and include withholding colostrum and giving substitute feeds for the first few hours or days (Morse et al 1990 [17]). In the past few decades, recommendations in the UK about the timing of the first breastfeed has ranged from waiting until six hours after birth (Myles 1975), to ensuring that the baby is fed within the first half hour after birth (WHO/UNICEF 1989).

Four randomised trials were identified which examined this question. They demonstrate that early contact combined with early breastfeeding can have beneficial effects on the latency to initiating the first breastfeed and weight gain in the first three days (Eppink 1969 [18]), on the relationship between the mother and her baby (Widstrom et al 1990 [19]), and on the baby's core temperature (van den Bosch and Bullough 1990 [20]). No impact on breastfeeding duration has been shown by the early initiation of breastfeeding (Salariya et al 1978 [21]), independent of feed frequency.

Eppink (1969) [18] allocated 60 babies alternately to be fed either within eight hours of delivery or to follow routine hospital care (24hr or more delay to initiating breastfeeding). The median latency to initiating the first breastfeed was shorter in the early contact group (30 sec vs 50 sec). Infant weight loss by day three was less in the experimental group (difference 1.25 oz, p<0.05), although these babies were deemed to need suctioning more often.

In Salariya's study (1978) [21], 111 women were randomised. In one group women were asked to breastfeed within the first 10 minutes, while those in the second group followed routine care, feeding between two and six hours after birth. The same women were also randomised to a 2-hourly or 4-hourly breastfeeding policy until lactation was established. The results indicated that the prevalence of breastfeeding at 6 and 12 weeks was affected neither by feeding early nor feeding frequently, although the authors suggest that women who fed both early **and** frequently had an increased duration of breastfeeding. On its own, feeding frequently was associated with an earlier initiation of milk production (see pages 33–35 below) while early feeding had no such effect on the initiation of production.

A study conducted in Thailand (Woolridge et al 1985 [22]) confirmed an absence of effect on the initiation of milk production; a 24hr delay in mother-infant contact and when the first feed was offered had no effect on milk output over the first five days post-partum. Despite the experimental intervention, however, the first feed did not take place until more than 4 hours after delivery, although once mother and baby were re-united there was a high level of mother-infant contact.

Widstrom and her colleagues (1990 [19]) randomised 57 primiparous women to either early contact and suckling within 30 minutes, or early contact and suckling according to the hospital routine which was approximately 8 hours following delivery. Although it appeared that the first attempts at breastfeeding were more successful in the later feeding group, examination of the relationship between mother and baby demonstrated that significantly more women in the early suckling group were talking to, and relating to their babies on the fourth day following delivery.

One randomised trial (van den Bosch and Bullough 1990 [20]) examined the effect of early feeding on the baby's core body temperature. One hundred and sixty mothers and their babies were randomised to two groups: in one group, they were encouraged to breastfeed as soon as possible following birth. In the other, they received 'normal management', where infants were placed in cots with a heated mattress and their mothers breastfed them when they were ready, usually after bathing and resting. Significantly fewer babies in the early sucking group had temperatures below 36.5°C at 8 a.m., and early skin-to-skin contact is recommended for all babies (whether breastfed or bottle-fed).

Several non-randomised prospective studies have also identified the benefits of early feeding (Johnson 1976 [23], Valdes et al 1993 [24], Righard and Alade 1990 [25], Prasad and Costello 1995 [26], de Chateau et al 1977 [27]).

The study by Johnson (1976) [23] was of only 12 women so is inconclusive.

Righard and Alade (1990 [25]) compared uninterrupted contact between mother and infant for at least one hour, versus immediate contact but with the baby then being removed for weighing and dressing. The results of this study should be treated with caution as the decision about which group the mother should be in was made by mothers and midwives. In the uninterrupted contact group 24 of the 38 babies 'sucked correctly' at the first feed compared to only 7 of the 34 in the separated group. Twenty six babies did not suck at all at the first opportunity to feed, in both groups; of these, 25 were born to mothers who had received pethidine.

Two studies evaluated an antenatal education intervention programme (Valdes et al 1993 [24], Prasad and Costello 1995 [26]) involving training of the multidisciplinary healthcare team. The healthcare team then instructed women in the benefits of early breastfeeding. In both studies the intervention group showed an increase in early initiation of breastfeeding and a reduction in the giving of supplementary feeds. Valdes et al (1993) showed that at 6 months exclusive breastfeeding was increased in the intervention group.

de Chateau and his colleagues ran three non-randomised controlled studies between 1972–1975 [27]. In one study, reported in 1977, 42 mothers were either encouraged to have immediate postpartum skin and feeding contact with their baby, or were allowed just a brief glimpse before their baby was taken away. The duration of breastfeeding was significantly increased in the early contact and feeding group.

In a study by Widstrom and her colleagues of routine gastric suctioning of the newborn (1987) [28], it was observed that in 10 babies, who did not receive suctioning, spontaneous sucking and rooting movements started to occur 15 minutes after birth, and reached a maximum at 45 minutes (sucking) and 60 minutes (rooting). The first hand to mouth movement was observed at a mean of 34 minutes, and the infants found the nipple and started to feed at a mean of 55 minutes. All of these behaviours were delayed by between 7–12 minutes in the 11 babies who received suctioning.

Discussion   Research demonstrates that no restrictions should be placed on contact between the mother and her baby at any stage, or on the time of the first breastfeed. Benefits identified from removing restrictions include an increased duration of breastfeeding, an enhanced relationship between mother and baby, and a reduction in the number of babies with temperatures below 36.5°C.

No research has demonstrated a 'critical period' for the first feed in terms of breastfeeding success, and there are therefore no grounds for restricting the mother's choice, or for interfering with the normal behaviour exhibited by the baby. One non-randomised study (Righard & Alade 1990 [25]), however, suggested that interrupting the period of contact, even though it was subsequently re-instated, impaired the tendency of the baby to initiate 'correct' feeding.

Although every woman should be given the opportunity to feed soon after birth, there is no evidence to suggest that if she does not feed immediately, she cannot establish effective breastfeeding, or that intimate skin-to-skin contact at a later stage may not be equally beneficial. Women who have a delayed onset to breastfeeding, therefore, should be reassured that this is not a contraindication to establishing breastfeeding successfully. They should be encouraged to have close and intimate contact with their baby after delivery even if breastfeeding is not possible, or at a later stage if such contact is not immediately possible (for example, due to obstetric or neonatal causes). For example, a review of skin-to-skin care (also known as kangaroo care) for preterm infants (Anderson, 1991) showed that the greatest impact of such an intervention was on the duration of breastfeeding.

One of the WHO/UNICEF's 'Ten Steps to Successful Breastfeeding' is to encourage women to breastfeed within the first half hour after birth (Taylor et al 1985, WHO/UNICEF 1989). In the UK, this Step has been revised in the light of evidence from Widstrom's et al's trial (1990 [19]) that some babies were unable to initiate breastfeeding in under 30 minutes, so attempts to do so with all babies would be unsuccessful in a proportion of cases, although they will still benefit from the early initiation of contact. Widstrom et al's earlier study (1987 [28]) indicated that babies demonstrate a range of times at which they are ready to feed, and that this behaviour can be disturbed by interventions. Strenuous attempts to feed the baby before he or she is ready could have a similar effect, and there is the further anxiety that hospital staff might apply the figure of 30 minutes prescriptively, rather than permissively. Instead, the evidence suggests that mothers and babies should have uninterrupted, close and intimate contact after birth. If this contact is skin-to-skin, and prolonged, then the baby will have free access to the breast and will be able to feed when he or she is ready.

The results of Righard and Alade's study (1990) suggest that this normal range of behaviour can also be interrupted by the use of pethidine for the mother in labour, and caregivers should be sensitive to the possible effects on the baby's ability to feed in the early hours and days after birth.

PRACTICE IMPLICATIONS:

- Early skin-to-skin contact between the mother and baby should be regarded as the norm (so long as circumstances allow it) and the benefits of this for all mothers and babies explained to all parents antenatally. This practice should be supported by hospital policy and offered as standard care by staff. Some women may not wish this and their wishes should be respected.

- The period of skin-to-skin contact should be prolonged, and should not be interrupted or curtailed by unnecessary procedures (e.g. gastric suctioning, weighing, or washing and wrapping the infant) unless the mother requests this.

- The opportunity to initiate the first breastfeed can be taken at this time, when both baby and mother show a natural readiness to feed.

- Professional assistance should be available to the mother at the first feed. Whilst this may provide the opportunity to offer specific education on breastfeeding technique, care should be taken not to interfere with the natural interaction between the mother and her newborn, or to overload her with information – the request for information should be mother-led.

- Women should be informed antenatally of the possible adverse effect that pethidine (given in labour) may have on the baby's ability to feed at this time (and in the subsequent hours and days after birth).

- There is little support however for a 'critical period' during which women must initiate breastfeeding. If the mother is motivated to breastfeed, then skilled sensitive support offered at subsequent feeds is likely to result in a beneficial outcome. If the initiation of breastfeeding is delayed for any reason, women should be reassured that having uninterrupted skin-to-skin contact at any stage later may be of equal benefit.

- Where oral Vitamin K is routinely administered to the newborn this should not immediately follow the first breastfeed (some time delay should ensue). This will help to ensure that, if the baby finds the oral preparation distasteful, there will be no association with breastfeeding, which might otherwise lead to breast refusal.

Further research   Further research is needed to describe the normal range of behaviour in mothers and babies who are allowed uninterrupted contact, in an environment which is supportive of breastfeeding; such research as exists has been carried out on very small numbers. Studies should describe the range of times after birth at which the mother is most likely to feel relaxed and ready to feed, and the baby is most likely to be receptive to feeding (as opposed to nuzzling at the breast). They could also describe the help that women need for this first feed to be effective. Examination of the range of normal behaviour would also help to inform the debate about how long babies should be allowed to sleep between feeds in the early days. There is anxiety about hypoglycaemia developing in babies in whom the first breastfeed is delayed (Hawdon et al 1993, Anderson et al 1993). Such anxiety may result in routine testing, or in testing babies who sleep longer than a defined period. Long periods of sleep may be a normal response to the trauma of birth, or may indicate the need for intervention.

The effects of different methods of pain relief in labour on the baby's ability to breastfeed should be studied.

Research is also needed to examine the relationship of the timing of the first feed with subsequent breastfeeding duration in situations where breastfeeding is delayed; for example, women who have a general anaesthetic, whose babies are sick, who are themselves ill, or who have cultural beliefs about the need to delay the onset of breastfeeding.

Prevention of sore nipples

Sore nipples and painful breasts are among the three commonest reasons women give for abandoning breastfeeding (along with 'insufficient milk' and 'baby would not suck/rejected breast'). Many of these problems would be prevented if the baby was enabled to feed without causing damage to the mother's nipples; achieving trauma-free feeding should also result in effective removal of milk, thereby alleviating the commonest problem of the three – 'insufficient milk'.

Positioning of the baby at the breast   Two different types of sore nipples were described by Gunther in 1945 [29]; an erosive or petechial lesion, and a fissure of the nipple. This paper was the first to ascribe severe pain and nipple damage to the position of the baby on the breast. This study also described the very high pressure exerted when a baby is at the breast but not able to obtain a good supply of milk, and showed an association between the incidence of soreness and the baby's birthweight.

A good understanding of the importance of the positioning of the baby at the breast was later gained from the cineradiographic studies by Ardran et al (1958), and ultrasound studies conducted by Smith et al (1985), Bosma et al (1990) and Weber et al (1986); this work was summarised by Woolridge (1986a). These studies demonstrate the relationship between the baby taking a good mouthful of breast tissue into his or her mouth, and the resultant lack of damage to the nipple with unrestricted milk flow. With good positioning of the baby at the breast, the nipple is protected from damage at the back of the baby's mouth, and the milk ducts under the areola are effectively milked by the baby's tongue. The result should be pain-free feeding, effective milk removal, and a satisfied baby.

Clinical research to examine practices related to these effects is limited, although initial results seem very promising. In one randomised trial carried out in Sweden (Righard and Alade 1992 [30]), 82 breastfeeding women were observed at 4–6 days after birth (by one observer) and 54 were identified as having an 'incorrect breastfeeding technique' ('nipple-sucking'). These 54 women were then randomised to one of two groups, either receiving instruction on how to correct 'nipple sucking' or not. Women identified as having a correct breastfeeding technique at discharge from hospital ('correct' and 'corrected' groups combined) were significantly more likely to be breastfeeding, both exclusively and partially, at four months after birth.

A pilot study by Duffy et al (1997 [31]) tested the effectiveness of an antenatal group session focused on teaching positioning and attachment. Although small, it suggested that a dedicated session of this nature was highly effective at reducing the incidence of nipple pain and trauma in the first four days post-natally; that women were better able to position and attach their babies; and that they were much more likely to be breastfeeding at six weeks. The limited nature of this study urges caution in generalising too much from these striking findings.

Long (1995), in a non-randomised study, implemented breastfeeding workshops designed to increase women's knowledge, skills and attitudes. The main reported benefit to mothers was an increase in their level of confidence postnatally, with higher numbers breastfeeding at 8–12 weeks.

Topical agents to prevent nipple pain

In the recent past a large range of substances have been advised for women to apply to their nipples in an effort to avoid damage and pain. A few of these have been examined in studies.

CHLORHEXIDINE SPRAY

A chlorhexidine aerosol spray has been used, sometimes as a routine measure, for the purpose of preventing sore nipples. One double-blind randomised controlled trial (Slaven et al 1988 [32]) of 723 women who were allocated either to receive chlorhexidine spray, or a placebo spray, found no differences in the incidence of sore or cracked nipples between the two groups of women. A similar placebo-controlled trial of 200 women (Herd and Feeney 1986 [33]) found an increase in the numbers of women in the placebo group who stopped breastfeeding in the first four weeks (31% vs 18% in the experimental group). The amount of nipple trauma experienced by women in the experimental group was increased, however. A small, non-randomised comparison of chlorhexidine spray with the use of expressed breast milk spread on the nipples after feeding found no differences between the two groups (Rickitt 1986 [34]).

OTHER TOPICALLY-APPLIED PREPARATIONS

A small, non-randomised prospective study of 20 women (Riordan 1985 [35]) examined the use of lanolin and tea bags. No significant differences were found.

One randomised controlled trial of 94 women compared the use of warm moist tea-bag compresses, warm water compresses, expressed breast milk, or instruction alone (Buchko et al 1993 [36]); all three treatment groups also received instruction. No significant differences were found, although there was some indication that warm water compresses were more effective than other means in the alleviation of any nipple pain developing during the course of the study.

Pugh et al (1996 [37]), in a follow-up to this study (Buchko et al 1993 [36]), dropped moist tea bag compresses from the trial as they had been associated with more nipple pain. Instead they included a lanolin product (USP-lanolin with pesticide residues removed), which they compared with warm water compresses, expressed breast milk with air drying, or breastfeeding instruction alone. A larger group of 177 women was studied, with all groups receiving an educational training plan in breastfeeding in addition to the allocated treatment. No significant differences were found in pain intensity or duration of breastfeeding.

Lavergne (1997 [38]) conducted a trial involving 65 women all of whom were already experiencing sore nipples. The study compared tea bag compresses, warm water compresses, or no compresses and found that both treatments were equally effective at reducing self-reported nipple pain. However, both the study design used and the recurrent self-rating of pain at each feed would be likely to encourage an effect of treatment over no treatment.

There has been increasing interest recently in the concept of 'moist wound healing' whereby a waterproof barrier (of sterile petroleum jelly or a proprietary lanolin formulation) is placed over the lesion (Hinman & Maibach 1963, Sharp 1992). This allows air to reach the wound but ensures moisture retention, so allowing granulation to form across the wound without it drying out. No controlled studies of adequate size have been published to date, although Spangler & Hildebrandt (1993) report reduced nipple pain in a group of 50 mothers using a proprietary lanolin product on days 6–10 after delivery. It is plausible that this process may have contributed to the previously reported claims by women that oil-based formulations (e.g. lanolin, 'Calendula', 'Kamillosan') are beneficial with nipple soreness.

EXPRESSED BREAST MILK

Breast milk has been found to contain 'epidermal growth factor' (EGF), principally demonstrated to promote growth of the gut epithelium (Read et al 1988), but potentially of therapeutic benefit by promoting the growth and repair of skin cells (Brown et al 1989). This is the reasoning behind the topical application of a small amount of expressed breast milk onto nipples which are sore or cracked and letting them air-dry in order to encourage skin growth and repair. Such a practice may benefit the repair of broken or damaged skin (cf. moist wound healing, cited above). Where, however, the soreness is caused by a topical yeast infection (*Candida albicans* / 'thrush') such a measure could be counter-productive as the lactose (milk sugar) would act as a substrate for growth of the yeast. Accurate diagnosis of the cause of nipple soreness if essential therefore, as appropriate treatment of a topical yeast infection would be to wipe away residual milk and saliva after the feed, possibly with an emollient, and to apply an anti-fungal agent topically. As cited above, however, the small study conducted by Rickitt (1986 [34]) showed no difference between expressed breast milk and chlorhexidine spray applied to the nipples.

Discussion   Painful breastfeeding is more commonplace in societies where prolonged exclusive breastfeeding is achieved only by a minority of women, and where breastfeeding in public is rare. Women have little opportunity to observe the simple tasks of how to sit comfortably for feeding, holding her baby so that he or she is offered the breast at an appropriate angle, and ensuring that her baby has a good mouthful of breast, for feeding not to hurt. In such societies it is hard for women to learn from each other. Caregivers in the UK, therefore, must become skilled at helping women learn to breastfeed, and to pass on the necessary expertise in a sensitive and supportive manner. This should involve ensuring that the baby has a good mouthful of breast, that the feed does not hurt the mother, and that milk flow is unimpeded.

No studies have found convincing evidence that any topical agents will help to prevent nipple pain. Such practices may detract attention from helping the mother to achieve a pain-free feed. It is also possible that the use of preparations such as lanolin and chlorhexidine may provoke a skin reaction in some women. There are no grounds for using topical agents to prevent nipple pain and, while the application of either expressed breast milk or a waterproof barrier to nipple cracks or lesions is theoretically supported, there are no adequate trials to date.

PRACTICE IMPLICATIONS:

- Professionals should be able to advise a mother on how to feed her baby effectively and without pain, and impart this knowledge antenatally. The criteria for establishing whether this requirement has been met are explained in Key Practice Area C.

- Professionals should also be able to identify attachment of the baby at the breast which fails to fulfill these criteria and recommend improvements in a way that the mother can implement herself.

- Professional assistance of this sort should be available to all women throughout the period of attendance by midwives and thereafter, through continued health professional or voluntary support.

KEY PRACTICE AREA B

Professional assistance with positioning and attachment

One key *Practice Implication* which recurs throughout this and subsequent sections is that accurate technical support and assistance with positioning and attachment of the baby at the breast should be accessible to all women, and such help should be delivered with care, skill and sensitivity. The acquisition by healthcare professionals of the necessary expertise, and gaining the experience to deliver these skills effectively to women, so enabling them to practice them for themselves, should be regarded as vital to ensuring a successful outcome for breastfeeding. As such this deserves special recognition as a *key area of professional practice*.

Healthcare professionals and other caregivers with responsibility for assisting women with the management of breastfeeding should possess:

- An up-to-date, soundly-based physiological knowledge of the anatomy of the breast, the mechanisms of milk secretion and the principles of 'suckling' (by which the baby secures milk from the breast).
- A sound understanding of what represents physiologically appropriate positioning and attachment, and an ability to recognise positioning which is causing pain or leading to ineffective milk removal.
- A working familiarity with how to assist mothers in achieving effective positioning and attachment, and how to correct a painful or ineffective technique.
- The skill to enable women to achieve effective positioning and attachment for themselves, consistently and reliably.
- Professional training should reflect this necessary mix of knowledge, skills and counselling ability essential to the effective provision of care and support to the breastfeeding woman in establishing pain-free, effective breastfeeding with her baby.

It is strongly urged that development of the knowledge and the skills to implement it become a mandatory requirement of midwifery pre-qualification training (for instance, as part of EU Midwives Directive (80/154–155/EU) or as an additional requirement of midwifery training and practice as set by the UKCC).

It is also implicit that appropriately skilled healthcare workers must be accessible to mothers in the postnatal period, especially midwives who are trained to help women with breastfeeding. Their workload must allow them sufficient contact time with mothers to enable them to pass on the necessary expertise required to breastfeed successfully.

KEY PRACTICE AREA C

Pain-free, effective feeding

Throughout this document we have used the phrase 'pain-free, effective feeding' quite explicitly to describe the ideal outcome of the breastfeeding in functional terms, rather than to qualify positioning and attachment as either 'good', 'correct' or 'adequate'. The latter terms imply a value judgement by the caregiver about the quality of the mother's breastfeeding, which may be discordant with what the mother is feeling or what her baby is experiencing. For instance, if a midwife were to describe a baby as 'well-positioned' or showing 'good attachment', yet the mother still found feeding painful, or her baby remained hungry and unsettled after feeds, then clearly the midwife's value judgement is incorrect.

When such words are used positively to describe what a mother is doing they can improve her self confidence and her self-belief that she is doing well, but only if that report is not at odds with what she is feeling (soreness and pain) or with what her baby is experiencing (hunger and distress). It is unfortunately the case that one person's view of what constitutes 'good fixing' can be substantially discrepant with that of a more experienced caregiver. Furthermore, the negative counterparts of these terms – 'bad', 'incorrect' or 'inadequate' – are prejudicial and when used to describe a woman's feeding technique, as they often are, their effect on her can be dispiriting and disempowering, reducing both her confidence in her ability to feed and her self-esteem.

We have therefore elected not to perpetuate use of terms which imply that a third party can make an accurate value-judgement about the quality of feeding. Instead, we have opted for a phrase which describes the functional outcomes of feeding as either satisfactory or unsatisfactory for both the mother and her baby. It remains necessary, however, to define in practical terms what we mean by each element of the phrase 'pain-free, effective feeding'.

Pain-free feeding is defined solely from the mother's perspective, and while it is recognised that there may be other causal factors contributing to nipple pain (e.g. a pathogenic agent, the topical application of a chemical agent, or an oral anomaly of the baby), most commonly, and ultimately, it is the baby's mouthing action at the breast which results either in trauma being delivered to the nipple and breast or the absence of trauma. Whether or not feeding is pain-free can only be established by asking the mother in an open-ended manner 'How does feeding feel?'; closed questions, such as 'Now, that doesn't hurt does it?', are inappropriate.

Effective feeding is defined primarily by outcomes for the infant (e.g. settled after feeds, growing adequately), but also by the avoidance of common breastfeeding ailments for the mother other than nipple pain (e.g. engorgement). An absence of pain or soreness does not automatically mean that feeding is effective.

continued overleaf

KEY PRACTICE AREA C

Pain-free, effective feeding

continued from previous page

- The baby feeds well with prolonged bursts of strong slow sucking interspersed increasingly with pauses as the feed progresses. The baby reaches a clear end-point for the feed, detaching him or herself from the breast. He/she remains settled for a period after a feed which is acceptable to the mother. Babies may become unsettled or cry after individual feeds in response to a variety of sources of discomfort (e.g. pain, wind, colic, isolation, loss of contact, cold) as well as to continuing hunger. If the baby is persistently unsettled this should be addressed by further attention to the feeding process and to the management of feeds. An inability to resolve recurrent bouts of distress may indicate the need to address parenting skills more generally.

- The infant is showing a reasonable or moderate increment in weight between successive weighings (1–2 weeks apart) and the trend taken across a series of such weighings is satisfactory. Healthcare professionals should be cautious not to upset a mother by carelessly reporting her baby's weight change: should a baby show an apparent failure, in a single week, to maintain the consistent weight gain shown over previous weeks, further weighings, on the same time-scale as before, are indicated to identify the long-term trend.

- The infant is producing several wet nappies per day and an appropriate number of bowel movements for his/her size; this could be from several small motions per day, to the occasional large evacuation every several days (so long as the baby is not distressed, the motions are not hard, or the baby constipated).

- The infant is of a healthy appearance (colour and skin tone), showing no signs of dehydration and be of a happy disposition for some/most of the time.

- Satisfaction with feeding should also be mother-led, so the basic pattern of feeds, both day and night, should be acceptable to the mother. If she finds either the length or the frequency of feeding unacceptable she should be offered assistance.

- The mother should not be experiencing milk retention or stasis, engorgement or any discomfort associated with retained milk or excessive milk production. The mother should not be experiencing recurrent bouts of non-infective mastitis.

Further research More studies, such as that by Duffy et al (1997), should focus on the content of antenatal teaching sessions to determine which qualitative aspects are most effective at improving the breastfeeding outcome for women (in terms of both increasing breastfeeding duration and reducing the prevalence of nipple pain). Issues such as who offers the training sessions, the enthusiasm with which they present information, who attends, their receptiveness to the information, the nature of the message, the content of the knowledge imparted, the emphasis placed on technical aspects of breastfeeding, on the importance of positioning and attachment, and the practical skills transferred, are all areas which need to be addressed.

There have been no studies examining either of how to train caregivers to help women to position the baby effectively, or of how caregivers can best teach women how to position their baby effectively at the breast. **Pain-free, effective feeding is fundamental to successful breastfeeding and research is urgently needed to examine training programmes for caregivers to educate them in this essential skill, and how best to impart this to their clients.**

Frequency and duration of breastfeeding

Until the last decade, it was common for babies to be fed 'by the clock', either every three hours or every four hours (Fisher 1986, Woolridge 1996). Although this practice has been changing (Garforth and Garcia 1989, White et al, 1992, Foster et al, 1997) many women and caregivers seem to be uneasy if the baby wishes to be fed much more, or much less often, than six or seven times a day.

Limiting the time that babies spend on the breast seems to have been motivated by a belief that this would protect women from developing sore nipples. Regimes of progressive increases in the time at the breast (two minutes each side on the first day, four on the second, and so on) imply that the mother's nipples will become used to feeding and will 'toughen' over time. Evidence for this theory, however, is absent.

There are likely to be adverse consequences associated with restricting feeding times. Physiological studies, for example, demonstrate that milk composition varies over the course of a feed (Hytten 1954, Woolridge and Fisher 1988), with the fat content increasing and the volume decreasing as the feed progresses. In theory, therefore, limiting feeding time could preferentially reduce the intake of fat, which led Woolridge and Fisher (ibid) to hypothesise that an imbalance could develop in the baby's volume intake relative to his/her fat or calorie intake. A range of symptoms can arise but progressive calorie restriction will lead to slow weight gain or even failure-to-thrive in the infant, while over-ingestion of lactose can result in symptoms of lactose malabsorption – colic, wind, and loose acid stools. The authors cite case studies in support of their theory and further evidence comes from studies which have shown raised breath hydrogen levels in 'colicky' babies (Moore et al 1988, Miller et al 1989), but evidence from clinical studies is lacking. The main practice recommendation arising from this study, however, was that the rigid expectation that both breasts would be offered at a feed should be replaced by a more flexible pattern by which the baby was encouraged to finish feeding from the first breast, before the second was offered; if the second breast were not required by the baby, this would be accepted by the mother and the caregiver. The publication resulted in a shift in professional practice, although sometimes as a result of misinterpretation it led to the undesirable imposition of a rigid one-breast only patterns on nursing couples.

The first study to examine the outcomes for babies fed on different regimes was carried out by Illingworth and his colleagues using a non-randomised comparison design in the early 1950s (Illingworth et al 1952 [39]). Two different hospital wards were used. In one ward, the policy was a 'self demand' feeding schedule; in the other, the ward policy was a rigid 4 hourly feeding schedule. One hundred and thirty seven breastfeeding women and their infants were studied. Outcomes measured included the baby's weight gain by the 9th day, engorgement and sore nipples. The results indicated that babies regained their birthweight significantly earlier, and there was a significant reduction in breast engorgement and sore nipples in the mothers who were in the 'self demand' feeding group (Illingworth et al 1952 [39]).

Mothers in one of the groups in Salariya's randomised controlled trial (1978) were asked to feed every two hours, while the other group was asked to feed every four hours. The results showed that the onset of lactation (assessed by palpation of the breast) occurred in a greater proportion of women in 48 hours or under if the infant fed 2 hourly rather than 4 hourly. The number of women breastfeeding at 6 weeks and 12 weeks was also slightly higher in the group that fed 2 hourly although this was not significant (Salariya et al 1978 [21]).

de Carvalho and his colleagues carried out a small non-randomised prospective study (1984) [40] in which women were asked to feed their babies either every 3–4 hours, or 'on demand'. No differences were found in nipple soreness between women in the two groups. There was a decrease in nipple soreness after day 6, in spite of a significant increase in the frequency and duration of feeds.

Infant weight gain also appeared to increase in babies fed frequently in a non-randomised experimental study by de Carvalho et al (1983) [41]. On day 15 after birth, babies in the frequent feeding group took significantly more milk and gained significantly more weight than infants fed on a 3 to 4 hourly regime (de Carvalho et al 1983 [41]). There were, however, pre-existing differences in birthweight between babies in the two groups which may have influenced this finding (babies in the experimental group were 478g heavier at birth on average than those in the control group).

One randomised trial failed to find any differences in weight loss and serum bilirubin levels in term infants fed three-hourly when compared to those fed four-hourly (Gale et al 1989 [42]). However, babies in the 3 hourly group only received two additional breast feeds daily for the first three days, and both groups supplemented the feed at 2 am with formula given by the nursing staff.

Two prospective studies concluded that babies feed for very different lengths of time if left undisturbed at the breast (Howie et al 1981 [43], Woolridge et al 1982 [44]). Both studies demonstrate that the length of a feed is a characteristic of the individual baby, and is a function of the rate of milk transfer from mother to baby – where there is a high rate of milk transfer feeds tend to be short in duration; conversely, feeds are prolonged if there is a slower rate of transfer. The latter study also showed that the rate of milk transfer is a characteristic both of milk release by the mother and the demand for milk by the baby. Both groups of authors suggest that women should be told about the highly individual nature of breastfeeding, and that they should be encouraged to feed their babies for as long as the baby wishes.

It is unclear what the normal feeding behaviour of a baby who is not subject to restrictions might be. There are very few reports in the literature of babies who are unsupplemented, and who have unrestricted access to the breast. Such reports as there are (Simsarian and McLendon 1942; Olmsted and Jackson 1950; Inch 1980; Hawken 1982; and de Carvalho et al 1983) suggest that babies may take as few as two feeds on the first day after birth gradually increasing to 15–17 feeds a day after day three, before then decreasing gradually. Yamauchi & Yamanouchi (1990), making natural observations on the incidence of breast feeds, showed that in the first 24 hours after birth the commonest number of feeds was 3 (range from 0–11), while in the second 24 hours the mode had increased to 7 (range 1–22).

Discussion Despite some equivocal data and the methodological weakness of certain studies, there is substantial evidence that the timing and duration of breastfeeds should be responsive to the needs of the baby. It appears that policies in the UK are for the most part based on 'demand feeding' (Garforth and Garcia 1989, White et al 1992, Foster et al 1997). Questions remain, however, about what advice women actually receive from caregivers and from their friends and family about what constitutes 'demand feeding', as the belief in limiting feeding time seems to be hard to change completely.

PRACTICE IMPLICATIONS:

- The attending health professional should establish whether the mother is happy with her baby's pattern of behaviour, and offer advice and support as and when required.

- Professionals will require training to gain the necessary skills in how to counsel women accordingly.

- No rigid advice should be given to new mothers concerning either the length or the frequency of breastfeeds. Flexible patterns of feeding should be encouraged, which are responsive to the baby's needs. Women should remain flexible about the pattern of feeds, as that desired by their baby (how often and how long) may change over time.

- Frequent feeds, unrestricted in length, will help the baby to secure the appropriate balance of fore- and hind-milk, and sufficient amounts of both.

- No rigid policy of offering one or both breasts should be imposed, instead the mother should be encouraged to find the pattern which suits her baby and which matches her milk supply.

- Unrestricted feeding cannot freely be practiced if the basic skills of positioning and attachment have not been acquired by the mother.

Further research   There are important questions which remain to be resolved about the range of normal behaviour in the days and weeks after birth. As mentioned in the previous section, there is concern, for example, that leaving a sleeping baby undisturbed for lengthy periods in the early days after birth will result in hypoglycaemia (Hawdon et al 1993, Anderson et al 1993). As a result, policies often stipulate that babies be woken after set periods and fed, to prevent this problem. Case reports suggest that sleeping for several hours may be quite normal (Olmsted and Jackson 1950), and under natural circumstances babies may feed as little as once or twice in the first 48 hours (Yamauchi & Yamanouchi 1990). Caregivers in the UK and elsewhere (Australia) are now leaving babies for very long periods between feeds in the early days, but further research is needed.

'Supplementing' the baby

The practice of giving breastfed babies additional feeds of formula, water, or glucose has been questioned in recent years, and while it is still widespread, evidence is that the practice is declining in the UK. The OPCS national survey in 1990 found that the proportion of breastfed babies who were given additional bottles in the first week of life had dropped from 50% in 1985 to 45% (White et al 1992). The most recent ONS survey has shown a further decline to 36% (Foster et al 1997), although this level remains unsatisfactory in the UK. In a large survey of professionals' views in the mid-1980s, reasons given for recommending additional feeds included thirst, jaundice and hunger (Garforth and Garcia 1989), either because breastfeeding was regarded as not yet established, or because it was thought to have failed.

Feinstein et al (1986) found an association between formula supplementation in hospital and a reduced likelihood of breastfeeding at 1 and 4 months, with the impact being most marked at 10 weeks of age. Kurinij & Shiono (1991) found an association between delays in the initiation of breastfeeding after delivery and the tendency to give bottles, from which they concluded that hospital practices

KEY PRACTICE AREA D

Professional assistance with flexible patterns of feeding

A further *Practice Implication* which recurs throughout this document is the encouragement of *frequent feeds* of *unrestricted length* and it is necessary to be quite explicit as to what they both imply.

Frequent feeding – Practice recommendation: The intervals between feeds are highly variable but show some individual specificity. Some babies will revisit the breast after a very short interval (15–20 minutes), but, during the daytime, intervals between feeds ranging from 1.5 to 4 hours are entirely normal. Intervals shorter or longer than this can be within the normal range, but if mothers find them unacceptable the healthcare professional should react sensitively to such anxiety by offering constructive advice.

Explanatory note: It is not uncommon to find a minimum number of 8 breast feeds per 24hr specified in some training manuals (particularly those used internationally, primarily for training unskilled field workers). This guideline is based on the observed association from population-based studies that larger milk volume intakes are associated with more frequent breastfeeds (Brown et al 1982, Girija et al 1984, Drewett et al 1989). From this it has been concluded that if a mother increases her feed frequency it will increase her milk volume; there is less direct evidence to support this assumption (Egli et al 1961, Drewett et al 1993). It remains the case, however, that if a mother offers too few feeds, by implementing unphysiological cultural practices (for example, by using a dummy to space feeds too far apart), this can lead to clinical consequences which are readily correctable by offering more frequent feeds.

It can still be inappropriate to impose this guideline in a prescriptive way with all women. So, while in population terms larger volume intakes *are* associated with higher feed numbers, on an individual basis the causal route may operate in reverse or not at all. For instance, a woman with an established high volume output (1 litre/day) may only feed her baby 4–6 times per 24hr; there is no need for her to feed more frequently. Conversely, the baby of a mother with a low milk output may be feeding 12–18 times per day; so it may either be the case that the mother is unable to comply if asked to feed more frequently, or, if she is able to comply, that it does not have the expected impact.

Nonetheless, it remains a sound general principle that flexible patterns of feeding mean frequent feeds; simply stated, the baby's opportunity to feed should not be limited by efforts to space feeds unnecessarily (for example, by imposing a 3–4 hour interval from the end of one feed to the start of the next where more frequent feeds are indicated).

continued overleaf

Professional assistance with flexible patterns of feeding

continued from previous page

Unrestricted feed length – Practice recommendation: Feed lengths are highly variable between babies, but individual babies tend to show a characteristic pattern. Evidence suggests that the length of a breastfeed is directly related to the rate of milk transfer, with babies taking short feeds (as short as 3–4 minutes) if there is a fast rate of milk transfer, and longer, more protracted feeds (45–60 minutes per breast) if the rate of milk transfer is slower (Howie et al 1981, Woolridge et al 1982). The rate of transfer generally increases as infants get older, so feed lengths should shorten, although babies may spend long periods on the breast for other reasons.

Explanatory note: A comparable argument surrounds the principle that feeds should be of unrestricted length. A baby who is ineffectively attached will feed interminably with little increase in the volume of milk secured. Feeds of unlimited length can only be advised for the baby who is effectively attached and well positioned at the breast. If this is not the case, unlimited feeding will predispose the mother to nipple pain and soreness. It is a pre-requisite, therefore, that if mothers are to be advised to offer the breast for an unrestricted period, they should already have been shown how to achieve trauma-free, optimal positioning and attachment of their baby at the breast and are able to implement the advice given.

Finally, feed length and feed frequency may be related. If feeds are commonly very long (over 40 minutes per breast) *and* the interval between feeds is short (20–60 minutes), the mother should be offered assistance by a skilled professional to ensure the mother is enabled to feed her baby effectively.

Patterns of feeding change dramatically in the early postnatal period, with few, relatively long feeds (as few as 1–2 feeds/24hr – Yamauchi & Yamanouchi 1990) being replaced by more frequent feeds of shorter duration (up to 12 feeds/24hr – ibid.) as milk production becomes established.

(such as a delay in the early initiation of breastfeeding) can promote formula use and so shorten breastfeeding duration indirectly.

Critics of the practice state that giving additional feeds interferes with the 'supply and demand' mechanism of milk production, and therefore reduces milk supply (McNeilly 1977, Daly et al 1993); that it interferes with the development of normal immunological mechanisms, thus reducing one of the primary benefits of breastfeeding (Matthew et al 1977); that it can result in allergic conditions in some babies (Host et al 1988, 1992); that it can cause reactive hypoglycaemia (Heck and Erenberg 1987); and that it causes 'nipple confusion' in the baby who may come to prefer feeding from a bottle, rather than feeding from the breast (Neifert et al 1995). It may also reduce the mother's confidence in her ability to breastfeed her baby without help (Neifert and Seacat 1987) and its use by hospital staff to settle the crying infant can establish a precedent which may become a model for future management of the unsettled infant when the mother returns home.

Descriptive studies of breastmilk intake in the first few days of life indicate that babies receive gradually-increasing amounts of colostrum and milk when allowed to feed according to their own needs (Houston et al 1983, Saint et al 1984, Casey et al 1986). Babies are able to regulate their own intake of breastmilk in terms of both quantity and quality, so even in hot climates they do not require additional fluids as they can regulate their feeding accordingly (Amroth 1978, Goldberg and Adams 1983, Brown et al 1986, Sachdev et al 1991).

There are two randomised controlled trials of the use of additional feeds in relation to serum bilirubin levels and the need for phototherapy in babies (Nicoll et al 1982 [45], Martinez et al 1993 [46]). Both trials were small (49 women in the study by Nicoll et al, and 125 women in that by Martinez et al), but they provided no evidence that babies who were unsupplemented were any more likely to need phototherapy, or to have a higher serum bilirubin level. Two non-randomised studies came to the same conclusion (de Carvalho et al 1981 [47], Johnson et al 1985 [48]).

The impact of routine fluid supplementation on breastfeeding outcome is the subject of a forthcoming lactation review in the Cochrane Pregnancy and Childbirth Module (protocol – Martin et al 1999), so will only be dealt with briefly here.

In one part of a three-part study (de Chateau et al 1977 [27]), the 'routine care' women received (involving test weighing and supplementation) was modified by discontinuing weighing before and after feeds, encouraging mothers that their own milk production was adequate and withholding supplementary fluids. Women receiving 'routine care' were six times more likely to stop breastfeeding in the first week after birth, and twice as likely to stop by the end of the second week (Winberg & de Chateau 1979).

Nylander et al (1993 [49]) conducted a before and after intervention study, which promoted early, frequent breastfeeds and the elimination of routine supplementation on a maternity ward. Although such a study design is methodologically weak (the possibility is not ruled out that secular changes in breast-feeding practice have affected the outcome rather than the intervention itself), this study is noteworthy as much for the scale of change in care produced by the intervention itself, as for the magnitude of the outcome produced; revealing just how pervasive systems of care based on routine supplementation had become.

The study was carried out with 407 women on the maternity ward of a large urban hospital in Norway. The most outstanding difference reported was in the ratio of breastmilk to supplementary fluid taken on day two. During the period of standard hospital care this was 20:80, with 100% of infants receiving a mean of 188 ml of supplementary fluid (sucrose or formula) [see Table 49], in contrast to 85:15 during the intervention period, with not more than 14% of babies receiving water and/or expressed breast milk as supplementation (amounting to 23 ml). This represents a dramatic shift in policy, from one of an almost complete reliance on routine supplementation when breastfeeding was delayed and limited in frequency, to one where this practice was virtually eliminated.

Increases in breastfeeding frequency produced by the intervention led to increase in breast milk intake of 58% (measured intake on day 2), although overall intake (including supplementary fluids) was reduced by 34%. In areas where this might raise clinical concern (incidence of hypoglycaemia or of hyperbilirubinaemia requiring phototherapy) significant differences were absent. Of the 12% of babies who, during the intervention period, were suspected of being hypoglycaemic (so were given expressed breast milk), none were confirmed to be so on blood glucose testing. Other outcomes were favoured by the intervention; a commonly recorded condition – "nausea" in the breast-fed baby – fell from 57% to 21% with withdrawal of supplementation with sugar solution. Babies in the intervention period lost more weight sooner (weight loss 6.4% by day 2.6, versus 4.6% by day 3.6 before the intervention), but regained their birthweight faster and were heavier than control infants by day 6.

Given the scale of impact on practice, the authors expressed some surprise at the seemingly low impact on measures of breastfeeding performance; the duration of exclusive breastfeeding was increased by one month, from 3.5 to 4.5 months. Nonetheless, from 1½ to 6 months of age, differences in the prevalence of exclusive breastfeeding significantly favoured the intervention (from 3 to 9 months for partial breastfeeding). It is clear, however, that even prior to the intervention the breastfeeding rates were demonstrably high.

Only two randomised controlled trials were found which examined routine use of bottles in the early days after birth (one involving formula, the other glucose water). Cronenwett et al (1992 [50]) evaluated the use of a single daily bottle feed of formula versus no additional bottle feed in 121 first time mothers who were committed to breastfeeding. They found no differences between the groups, although such a finding cannot be generalised to the use of frequent 'top-ups' by women with low confidence in their milk supply.

In a study by Martin-Calama et al (1997 [51]), conducted in a hospital implementing the 'Baby Friendly Hospital' principles, approximately half of the 180 mothers in the sample were permitted to give glucose water if their baby was unsettled after breastfeeding; the frequency and amount given was not recorded. All mothers were encouraged to practice baby-led feeding. There was a greater weight loss in the first 48hr after birth in the babies who did not receive glucose water, but by three days of age this was no longer significant and their subsequent weight gain was higher. There were differences in the mean body temperature, the number of episodes when maximum temperature was above 37.5°C, the blood glucose level in the first 24hr, and the number of episodes when blood glucose was detected below 2.2 mmol/l, all of which appeared adverse in respect of the unsupplemented babies. None of these, however, were regarded as having clinical significance for the well-being of the babies and no babies developed clinical symptoms. Breastfeeding was of significantly greater duration in the unsupplemented group (p<0.01), with significantly more mothers having introduced formula by one month of age (p<0.05) in the supplemented group [51].

Two non-randomised controlled clinical studies examined routine supplementation versus restricted supplementation (Houston et al 1984 [52], Gray-Donald et al 1985 [53]). Neither found significant differences between babies who were routinely supplemented and those who were not.

In the study by Gray-Donald et al (1985 [53]) the intervention involved restricting supplementation on one ward, while adhering to standard care on another. In particular, this meant that mothers on the restricted supplementation ward were woken at 2 a.m. to give a breastfeed, instead of the routine which was to give formula at this time (during the pre-trial period formula intake amounted to an average of 49 ml/dy for each baby). Bottles of glucose water, however, remained freely available on both wards in which the study was conducted (babies receiving 45 ml/day on average).

Houston et al (1984) identified differences between women from different social class backgrounds. In her study, women from social classes III, IV and V breastfed for longer if they were in the group which was encouraged to demand feed and to give supplements if they or the staff thought it was necessary, when compared to a group where supplementation was routine, or where it was restricted.

One survey of supplementary feeding practice in the maternity ward (Blomquist et al 1994 [54]) found that the risk of not being breastfed was three and a half times higher in babies who were supplemented.

Discussion   There is no evidence that routine use of additional fluids – water, glucose, or formula – is necessary to prevent jaundice, or to add to the baby's nutritional intake. There is some evidence that giving additional feeds to babies will reduce the duration and/or period of exclusivity of breastfeeding, without any compensating benefit, although the quality of individual studies is not strong. In particular, studies have not evaluated separately the impact of giving formula from offering bottles *per se*, whether they contain water, glucose or formula. So, in terms of the potential routes by which bottles might disrupt the breastfeeding process, little progress has been made towards evaluating the causes. There is also some evidence that particular groups of women may be more responsive to permissive patterns of care, rather than to ones which are essentially restrictive.

PRACTICE IMPLICATIONS:

Hospitals / Maternity Facilities:

- Healthcare facilities should ensure that they have a policy for supplementation of breastfed babies which is clear, up-to-date, evidence-based and which takes account of the possible adverse impact of giving supplements other than breastmilk for non-medical reasons.

- The policy should include guidelines which set out objective criteria for determining which babies are at risk (i.e. *not* healthy, term infants), and the circumstances when term babies may be placed at medical risk if they were not to receive supplementation.

- The policy should be widely available to staff within the facility, which should also monitor adherence to the policy by its staff. This should include recording instances of, and the reasons for, supplementing breastfed babies – this is a key item which should be routinely monitored.

- Professionals working within the healthcare facility should personally ensure that they are familiar with and adhere to the guidelines of that facility as they relate to the medical indications for supplementation.

- Professionals will need to develop their clinical skills for recognising normal, healthy infants, in order to reassure mothers whose infants are not in need of supplementation.

- The breastfeeding rate should be routinely audited as one of the key outcomes of the policy. Policy refinement should take place, as a routine part of the audit cycle, but can only be achieved by monitoring relevant outcomes over time.

- Professionals should gain familiarity with the issues of: (i) what fluid is appropriate for supplementation (e.g. manually expressed colostrum, expressed breast milk or formula), and (ii) by which route it is preferable for such fluids to be administered (e.g. naso-gastric tube, syringe, cup, spoon or bottle) – (see page 44).

Health professionals and caregivers:

- When working with mothers and their babies health professionals and other caregivers need to acquire certain essential skills in order to overcome apparent crises of milk supply without resorting to artificial supplementation.

- Professionals should evaluate each mother/baby pair individually when providing practical help to the mother.

- Professionals should be able to reassure the mother over most of the common concerns she might have about her milk supply, stressing that most are transient in nature and easily remedied.

- Encouraging the mother to be responsive with her pattern of feeding and to observe sound breastfeeding technique will overcome most crises of confidence in her milk supply.

- Professionals can also help to alleviate the common misinterpretation that infant crying and distress are due solely to 'under-feeding'.

- Practical assistance should include ensuring that the baby has effective access to the milk which the mother is producing.

Further research   There is insufficient research to guide practice in making decisions about which babies may genuinely need additional feeds. Further research is needed to address important questions such as:

- When should a baby's milk intake be deemed inadequate for his or her physiological needs?
- What level of weight loss in the baby should result in supplementation?
- When should a mother be encouraged to express milk in addition to breastfeeding?

Without this information, caregivers will face conflicts in making decisions about when to advise a mother to resist pressure to supplement routinely, while reassuring her that all will be well, versus a necessary decision to give additional feeds to a baby who is not receiving an adequate intake from the breast.

There are also questions which need to be addressed about women's views of this issue.

- Do women from different cultural backgrounds and social class groups have different views on whether or not they would like to give additional feeds to their babies?
- If so, what are these views and the beliefs that underlie them?
- Would some women prefer to give a bottle on a regular basis, to prepare for going back to work, or to feel that they are able to leave the baby with another caregiver for a few hours?
- Do some women feel reassured to know that their baby would take a bottle if necessary?

Methods of giving additional fluids

There has been debate in recent years about the possibility that giving feeds by bottle to breastfed babies either in addition to, or instead of, the breast may give them an artificial sucking experience which is counter-productive to the successful establishment of breastfeeding. The debate arose from the recognition of the different sucking techniques used while breast and bottle feeding (Bu'lock et al, 1990), although several descriptions in textbooks are contradictory (Eiger & Olds 1987 p24, Woessner et al 1987 p77) and have not been verified by imaging studies. Evidence from clinical trials is absent, however, for the syndrome which has come to be described as 'nipple confusion' (Neifert et al 1995). One paper describes the syndrome, and suggests that until the necessary research is carried out, it would seem prudent for caregivers to 'identify newborns at risk of nipple confusion and to minimise the use of bottle feeding in such babies' (Neifert et al 1995). There is no evidence available as yet to assist in such identification.

The use of 'cup feeding', whereby infants are fed from a small plastic cup, as an alternative to bottle feeding for babies who require additional fluids, has been increasing in recent years, in an effort to avoid nipple confusion. Descriptive studies of the effect of this practice have been carried out in neonatal and transitional care units, with babies who are small or sick.

Only one study, a randomised controlled trial, has examined this issue in term babies (Schubiger et al 1997 [55]). This trial, carried out with 602 women in Switzerland, examined the restriction of fluid supplements to healthy term infants (n=294) in the first five days after birth (compared with 308 control infants). Supplements of tea or formula, where given, were by cup or spoon as the alternative to the bottle (pacifier use was also restricted). There were no significant differences in the prevalence of breastfeeding at two, four or six months after birth, indicating that the use of bottles, *per se*, had not adversely affected breastfeeding rates. The experimental protocol with respect to bottle use, however, was violated in 39% of cases; of the remaining 180 infants, 92% received supplements of either dextrin-maltose or formula (equivalent figures for the control group were 5.5% and 97% respectively). These data suggest that one of the declared aims of the intervention, the restriction of fluid supplements (whether or not given by bottle), was not effectively implemented; this may be viewed as having reduced the potential of this study to evaluate the impact of withholding bottle teats and pacifiers on breastfeeding duration.

Discussion Given the strength of feeling among caregivers about the dangers of 'nipple confusion', there is a surprising lack of evidence to describe this condition, it's prevalence or it's treatment (caregivers sometimes even recommend passing a naso-gastric tube rather than give a bottle). Babies who are successfully breast-fed have also been observed to refuse bottles, suggesting that this is a general principle rather than something which only applies to babies who refuse the breast once exposed to bottles; the term 'acquired teat preference' has been coined to accommodate this (Woolridge 1996).

- Bottles and teats are interventions and should be recognised as such (See Key Practice Area E). Any intervention has the potential to cause harm if used routinely or in the wrong situation, and the potential to help if used sensibly and in the full knowledge that their artificial nature may disrupt a natural process.

- In consequence, professionals should review their practices concerning alternative methods for giving additional fluids and audit relevant outcomes. Individual circumstances should be carefully considered when selecting particular methods. For example, is the impact of bottles likely to be different if they contain mother's own expressed breast milk (MOBM) or artificial formula; will supplements be given during the establishment of lactation when their impact may be significant (as opposed to being offered for social reasons once breastfeeding is established when their impact is likely to be minimal).

- Professionals should ensure they are appropriately trained in alternative methods of supplementation to be employed (e.g. cup, spoon, syringe or tube feeding).

- Instruction on the appropriate use of alternative methods should also be given both to mothers, and to their partners, who can be expected to use such methods.

Further research   In the light of the possible adverse effects of withholding bottles from babies who might need additional fluids, a number of important question needs to be addressed.

- Are some term babies more likely to develop problems feeding at the breast than others?
- Can babies at risk of having their breastfeeding disrupted be identified?
- To what extent is cup feeding a suitable and acceptable alternative?

Use of pacifiers (dummies) with breastfed babies

The use of pacifiers to settle, soothe or otherwise occupy a fretful or distressed baby has become a widespread cultural practice. Documented reasons why mothers adopt the practice include: they are more sensitive to their baby's crying than mothers who don't use them; they use pacifiers either to space breastfeeds (perceived as being too frequent) or to reduce breastfeeds in number, as an active element of the weaning process (Victora et al 1997).

The use of pacifiers, however, has been implicated in several adverse outcomes including: increased risk of otitis media (Uhari et al 1996, Watase et al 1998), of oral candida infection (Darwazeh & al-Bashir 1995), reduced intellectual attainment (Gale & Martyn 1996, Barros et al 1997), reduced jaw muscle activity (Sakashita et al 1996) and greater incidence of abnormal jaw development (Ogaard et al 1994).

The prevalence of pacifier use differs by country, however, with rates of use among specified groups as high as 68% in the US (Howard et al 1999), compared with 24% in Norway (Arnestad et al 1998); the figure for a comparable group in the UK is 52% (Fleming et al 1996). Differential rates between women who breastfeed and women who bottle-feed have also been reported; in New Zealand, for example, they are 9% & 19% respectively (Mitchell et al 1993).

Avoidance of the use of pacifiers on maternity units is one of the global criteria by which hospitals are assessed for designation as 'Baby Friendly'. Simply stated, the criterion seeks to prevent healthcare staff from introducing pacifiers to individual women, and for this to be mandated within the hospital policy applying to all healthy term newborns. This recognises that the mother herself, or relatives and friends, may introduce the practice, but that healthcare professionals should not do so. There is a paucity of trials in this area, however, making it difficult to cite adequate evidence to resolve the debate surrounding their use.

Righard and Alade (1997) re-analysed data from a previous study (Righard & Alade 1992 [30]) to examine the association of 'incorrect nipple sucking' with pacifier use. At four months of age the prevalence of breastfeeding among women who used a pacifier with their baby was 44% compared with 91% among the group who did not use a pacifier. In the original study however, group allocation was not carried out with respect to pacifier use, so the result may reflect self-selection by the mothers (Righard & Alade 1992).

Righard (1998 [56]) reported a case-control study in which 52 mother-infant pairs with breastfeeding problems were compared with 40 without breastfeeding problems. The author, in an unblinded assessment, attributed 94% of the problems to an incorrect pattern of 'nipple-sucking', compared with 10% in the control group without breastfeeding problems. Seventy three percent of the study group used a pacifier compared with 30% in the control group. Neither of the studies, however, can resolve whether use of a dummy is integral to development of the problem, or whether the problem itself provokes the mother to use a pacifier as part of her attempt to overcome that problem.

Vallenas & Savage (WHO 1998) have reviewed epidemiological studies, conducted in Brazil (Victora et al 1993 & 1997, Barros et al 1995). These studies have controlled for confounding variables and shown that the greater the intensity of pacifier use, the greater the likelihood that breastfeeding will be of shorter duration; this 'dose-response' effect is suggestive of a causal link.

Discussion   To date, no prospective randomised controlled trial has been conducted to explore whether the use of bottle teats, and/or pacifiers (dummies) have a deleterious impact on the establishment of lactation. There remains widespread concern among clinical practitioners that their use is a practice with the potential to cause harm during the time when the mother is initiating and establishing lactation with her newborn.

Based on the studies cited here, it may be concluded that pacifiers are a contributory factor in the causal process leading to a shortened duration of breastfeeding. However, simply eliminating their use will not resolve the anxieties of the mothers who are most likely to employ them. A crucial element of any programme which discourages the use of pacifiers, must be efforts to build the mother's confidence in her ability to nourish, soothe and settle her breastfed baby through her own efforts.

Recent epidemiological data has suggested an association between pacifier use and a reduced risk of sudden infant death syndrome (SIDS) (Mitchell et al 1993, Fleming et al 1996). Until such time as this association is clarified, and/or the route by which it operates has been elucidated, hospital policy should state that pacifiers should not be permitted to interfere with the initiation and establishment of breastfeeding.

PRACTICE IMPLICATIONS:

- Practitioners should remain aware that pacifiers (dummies) represent an artificial intervention, with the potential to disrupt the initiation and establishment of lactation if introduced and used routinely at this time (See Key Practice Area E).

- There is adequate evidence available (predominantly epidemiological) to suggest that pacifiers (dummies) have an adverse impact on the duration of lactation and are associated with health problems. Healthcare staff should not, therefore, introduce the use of pacifiers to mothers and babies.

- Professionals should review both their policy and practice concerning the use of pacifiers on maternity units (the routine availability of pacifiers on maternity units implies endorsement of the practice by healthcare staff).

- Pacifier use should be audited (who introduced them, for what purpose, what is the outcome of breastfeeding for that mother), not just in hospital, but in the long-term.

- Where a mother (or her relatives/friends) introduces pacifiers onto the ward, dialogue should take place between the midwife and the mother in her care, with the aim of explaining the potential harm that pacifier use may have on the successful establishment of lactation, so that the mother is enabled to make a choice which is both free and informed.

- Professionals must possess the knowledge and skills necessary to determine the causes which lead a baby to being unsettled, in order to be able to help the mother overcome them without resorting to a pacifier.

- Professionals should also be able to advise the mother on a range of strategies to help her cope with a fretful or distressed infant (holding positions, baby massage, rocking and carrying, and/or changes to the baby's environment). The possession by parents of such therapeutic options is essential to successful parenting, not just to successful breastfeeding.

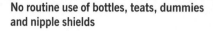

No routine use of bottles, teats, dummies and nipple shields

Bottles, teats and related devices should be recognised as **interventions** which are artificial in origin and nature. Whether they are used wisely or foolishly, routinely or as one-off use, like any intervention, they have the potential to cause harm.

Healthcare professionals have an obligation to minimise the use of any and all interventions that have the potential to cause harm, and maximise those that ensure a good breastfeeding experience for both the mother and her baby. Furthermore, it is essential that the potential risks associated with any intervention be discussed with the mother (parents) and her (their) informed consent sought before it is used. There should be no difference in procedure whether the intervention has been introduced by a member of healthcare staff (a supplementary bottle of formula, for example), or by the mother (use of a dummy brought into hospital by the mother, her relative or a friend).

In the absence of evidence to support or counter the concept of 'nipple confusion', decisions about the method of feeding babies who cannot feed from the breast are challenging. Professionals should assess each case on its merits, considering for example:

* the number of times/length of time for which the baby will need to be fed like this – is it only one feed, or is it likely to be the main method of feeding for several days or weeks?
* is the baby in need of satisfying oral experience that cannot be met in other ways? For example, for a baby in an incubator who is deprived of other forms of physical contact (cuddling, stroking) sucking may be very important. There is, however, no evidence to date on the relative merits of providing sucking experience to a baby on the short term versus depriving the baby of this, or its potential to disrupt the establishment of breastfeeding on the long-term.

So, in the absence of such evidence, there is an immediate and ongoing priority to audit use of bottle teats and pacifiers with babies and the subsequent outcome for breastfeeding with such babies and their mothers.

Nipple shields: Studies of nipple shields have shown them to reduce milk transfer from the mother to her baby. Widespread clinical experience suggests that they offer no greater assurance of breastfeeding success, but more than this, their routine use can contribute to the failure of breastfeeding. In contrast, clinical practitioners report individual successes when nipple shields are used judiciously. In such circumstances, however, they are an adjunct to the intrinsic skills of the practitioner, and the lactation is managed through to a satisfactory conclusion, a process which, ideally, should include withdrawal of the nipple shield.

Methodological bias cannot be excluded from such reports, however (e.g. subjective or selective case reporting), and so these reports should not modify the exclusion of nipple shields from **routine** postnatal care.

An individual practitioner taking responsibility for introducing use of a nipple shield with a mother and her baby, should also take responsibility for the eventual withdrawal of use of that shield. If that responsibility is to devolve to another person (professional or lay) then its introduction should not be considered.

Further research There are still circumstances where it remains routine for babies to be offered bottle-teats and/or pacifiers – on neonatal units, for example. There is still scope, therefore, to conduct a randomised controlled trial of the impact that teats and pacifiers may have on the initiation and establishment of lactation. Preterm babies remain one of the groups with the lowest breastfeeding rate and whether the routine use of teats/pacifiers contributes to this situation is not known.

To determine whether there are adverse effects of withholding pacifiers from babies who have no other form of oral stimulation (babies on neonatal units without ready access to their mother), several questions should be addressed by research.

- Are some term babies more at risk of develop feeding problems while breastfeeding than others and, if so, how can they be identified?
- Are there measurable indicators to establish whether babies deprived of pacifiers suffer emotional disadvantage or functional impairment that might not be averted by alternative oral strategies (earlier introduction of breastfeeding, use of cup-feeding for supplements).
- In how many cases is use of a pacifier the only successful therapeutic strategy for calming a fretful, distressed or unsettled baby? How commonly is it the case, in such circumstances, that his/her primary nutritional needs can be shown to have been adequately met?

Giving discharge packs of formula

Eight randomised trials were identified which examined the practice of giving packs containing formula and bottles to breastfeeding women when they leave hospital (Bergevin et al 1983 [57], Frank et al 1987 [58], Evans et al 1986 [59], Feinstein et al 1986 [60], Dungy et al 1992 [61], Snell et al 1992 [62], Bliss et al

1997 [63], and Dungy et al 1997 [64]), including a total of just under 3,500 women and babies. This topic is the subject of a forthcoming lactation review in the Cochrane Pregnancy and Childbirth Module (protocol – Donnelly et al 2000) and so will only be dealt with briefly in this review.

Studies varied as to whether the free formula sample was simply absent from the packs given to the experimental group [57, 59, 60 & 62], or whether its absence was offset by the provision of educational materials and breast pads [58] or replaced by a breast pump (hand) [61, 63, 64]. The outcome measure also differed being the proportion of babies either breastfeeding at all, or being breastfed exclusively at particular time points (from 1 week to 4 months).

Three studies showed either that breastfeeding duration was increased when the formula sample was absent (the greatest difference being detectable at around 3 months post-partum in the study by Frank et al [58]) or that fewer women had switched to bottle-feeding by a particular time post-partum (at three weeks in the study by Snell et al [62]). The remaining five studies were neutral, demonstrating no significant impact on the incidence of breastfeeding of receiving free formula samples in discharge packs.

Studies were more likely to be equivocal, however, where the presence of any breastfeeding *per se* was the outcome; when the outcome was the exclusivity of breastfeeding, several studies showed that babies were far more likely to be supplemented with formula in the groups receiving commercial discharge packs containing formula.

The two studies by Dungy and colleagues [61 & 64] reached conclusions which differed from each other; they attribute this to the fact that the first study was conducted with a population which was more vulnerable to free samples; their second study was conducted with a more middle-class, white population with a higher initiation rate for breastfeeding. A greater impact on populations of women, potentially more vulnerable to free samples, was also suggested by the studies of Bergevin et al [57] and Snell et al [62].

No study reported whether women were asked directly whether or not they gave their baby the free sample of formula contained in the pack, or for those women not receiving packs but who gave formula, from where they secured their formula. These factors may be relevant in the culture where most of these studies were conducted, where there is such ready access to formula. One study conducted in a developing country setting (Guthrie et al 1985) showed no apparent effect, although subsequent re-analysis of the data (Perez-Escamilla et al 1994) suggested that women who received a free sample of formula were less likely to breastfeed during the first 8 months after birth.

A randomised trial of gift packs containing formula amongst adolescent women, conducted by Neifert et al (1988 [65]), provided no data on outcome by treatment group by which to evaluate the impact of the free formula samples, although the authors reported no significant difference either in the duration of breastfeeding or the age at which formula supplementation was introduced.

Discussion   There is convincing evidence that giving packs containing formula and bottles to women at discharge from hospital increases the likelihood that babies will be supplemented with formula, and some evidence that it significantly decreases the duration of breastfeeding; such packs should not therefore be given to women. Giving packs containing a breast pump may be a way to give breastfeeding women a gift that does not compromise their chances of continuing to breastfeed.

PRACTICE IMPLICATIONS:

- The practice of giving discharge packs containing samples of formula has been discontinued in the UK and, based on the evidence, there would seem sufficient reason to maintain this position.

- Discharge information booklets can be recommended if they contain: (i) information on the health gains from exclusive breastfeeding until 4–6 months of age, (ii) up-to-date, soundly-based advice on how to avoid and overcome common problems of breastfeeding, (iii) advice on how to sustain exclusive breastfeeding until the time when weaning foods can be introduced, and (iv) guidance on sustaining breastfeeding beyond this point.

- Such information booklets should be free from any bias which might encourage women to switch from breastfeeding to artificial feeding, free from any commercial advertising, and should contain appropriate information as specified by regulation 21(1) of 'The Infant Formula and Follow-on Formula Regulations 1995' (UK SI 1995 No.77).

Further research   Further research is needed to help to identify the information and products which might help women to continue to breastfeed (e.g. self-help leaflets (hand expression, low milk supply), a simple hand breast pump).

5   Common breastfeeding problems

Five successive national surveys (Martin 1975, Martin & Monk 1982, Martin & White 1988, White et al 1992, Foster et al 1997) have each shown the most common reasons women report for stopping breastfeeding to be: sore nipples and breasts (30% of those who stopped in the first week), mothers feeling that they have 'insufficient milk' (35% of those who stopped in the first week, rising to 60% of those who stopped between 2 and 6 weeks), and feeling that the baby would not suck, or that he or she rejected the breast (25% of those who stopped within the first week). The reported incidences have also been rank-ordered in very much the same way with each successive survey.

It is of course likely that these reasons reflect only part of the story. Breastfeeding problems are often multifactorial, and women will describe a sequence of events leading up to their decision to stop in which physical factors interrelate with psychological factors and the support or otherwise that they receive (Houston 1984). They may also experience a number of different problems at the same time, such as sore nipples, engorgement, and anxiety about the baby getting enough milk. It is likely, therefore, that women's reasons for stopping are more complex than can be recorded in large postal surveys such as those undertaken by OPCS and ONS.

Problems may or may not lead to discontinuation of breastfeeding. Even a well motivated and well supported mother will find sore nipples and a crying baby challenging, and the more severe the problem, and the more problems she has, the more likely it will be that she will consider stopping altogether. If she does continue in spite of problems, she may feel she needs to give supplements to her baby, and it is likely that she and her immediate family will find that the problem disturbs many aspects of their lives, such as sleep and the ability to relax, go out, or enjoy the new baby.

This section will examine prevention and treatment of common breastfeeding problems. They fall into three main categories: sore nipples and breasts; problems with milk flow such as engorgement and mastitis; and problems with milk supply, such as 'insufficient milk', and an inconsolable baby.

5.1 Sore nipples and breasts

Sore nipples

The evidence related to the prevention of sore nipples resulting from positioning problems was described above on pages 26–29. It is likely that the majority of sore nipples could be prevented and treated by effective, pain-free positioning of the baby at the breast.

Some conditions may make this process more complicated, such as tongue-tie in the baby. This issue will be examined on pages 84–85.

The following studies have examined ways of treating sore nipples.

Nipple shields

Rubber or plastic 'nipple shields' are sometimes recommended to help women continue to breastfeed when they have sore nipples. These are placed over the nipple and held in place while the baby feeds. Critics of these shields suggest that milk volume will be decreased with their use, as they decrease the amount of nipple stimulation from the baby's mouth.

Woolridge et al (1980b) [66] compared milk flow and sucking patterns in women who used a commonly-available type of nipple shield (the 'Mexican Hat', so called because of it's distinctive shape), with a shield they developed for research purposes, made of a thin latex rubber. For the group of 16 women using the Mexican Hat shield, milk transfer to the baby was significantly reduced, and sucking patterns were affected. Use of the thin latex shield also reduced milk transfer, but not to such a great extent, and sucking patterns were unaltered. Auerbach (1990) [67] studied 25 women using the breast pump with two types of thin silicone rubber nipple shield, one modified to have a single large central hole. She found large reductions in milk volume with the use of both shields.

A randomised trial of 90 women in Australia (Nicholson 1985 [68]) compared the use of a nipple shield with either continued breastfeeding on the affected side or discontinuation of feeding until the damage had healed. No differences were found between the groups.

The same author carried out a descriptive study of women using nipple shields (Nicholson 1993 [69]), and found no difference in breastfeeding duration among women who used nipple shields and those who did not.

Breast shells

Breast shells are sometimes recommended to promote healing of sore nipples. These are hard plastic rounded cone-shapes, inserted inside the bra and worn between feeds to keep clothing away from the sore nipple. They are removed for feeding.

Only one small study has examined their use (Gosha and Tichy 1988 [70]). This study examined a shell which was designed with several small holes to allow free circulation of air. No differences were found between those who used them and those who did not.

Dressings (and other applications)

A small study, involving 50 women, conducted by Ziemer et al (1995 [71]), compared the benefit of a polyethylene film dressing applied to one breast, with the other breast acting as control. No differences existed in visually detectable damage, although women rated their pain intensity as lower with the film dressing (by 0.28 of a point, measured on a 5 point scale).

As previously discussed (page 28) studies of the use of lanolin, to form a semi-permeable waterproof barrier over lesions of the nipple (Riordan 1985 [35], Pugh et al 1996 [37]), have proved inconclusive.

Infection

Infection of the nipple can cause irritation and inflammation, with symptoms ranging from severe pain to itching and burning sensations. Such infections are not always identified. One paper reported 20 case studies where collaboration between a lactation consultant and a dermatologist was used to address persistent sore nipples (Huggins and Billon 1993 [72]). Women were assessed by the dermatologist and treatment included anti-fungal, antibiotic and steroid treatments applied topically. Eighteen of the twenty women referred showed improvement.

Amir and Pakula (1991) describe two case studies of women with candida. The symptoms of candida infection which they describe included persistent sore nipples and severe shooting breast pain. The pain resolved with topical miconazole and oral nystatin, although the latter is not supported theoretically as the absorption of nystatin is too low to reach therapeutic systemic levels (information from manufacturer). Tanguay et al. (1994) describe a series of 27 cases referred to a breastfeeding clinic and note the association with vaginal candidiasis, previous antibiotic use and nipple trauma.

Sore breasts

In many studies, sore breasts and nipples are presented together in the analysis (for example, White et al 1992). Women, however, experience pain in the breast as well as pain in the nipples, which may or may not be related. No studies have been identified which address the prevalence, prevention or treatment of sore breasts caused by factors other than engorgement and mastitis. Even in the absence of engorgement and mastitis, breast pain can occur during and between feeds. Suggested causes include spasm of the ducts, persistent reaction to nerve trauma, deep candida infection, and prolactin-induced mastalgia.

Discussion The primary treatment for sore nipples is to ensure that the baby has a good mouthful of breast tissue so that feeding does not hurt and nipple damage is able to heal (see Key Practices B – p26, and C – p27).

There is little evidence to inform practice in relation to other causes of sore nipples – for example, eczema, impetigo, dermatitis, or even the contact sensation of a well-positioned baby feeding at the breast, which individual women may perceive as pain. Practices based on clinical experience and a theoretical analysis of the problem have developed. These include the use of anti-fungal preparations for candida, and steroid preparations for dermatitis. But identification of women most at risk of developing these problems, accurate diagnosis, and the best regimes for treatment, are based on very little information.

The problem of breast pain, which some women describe as severe, has not been examined in any studies we identified.

PRACTICE IMPLICATIONS:

- The majority of common breastfeeding problems can be overcome by the simple application of basic physiological principles and a sound knowledge of how to implement practical guidance on positioning and attachment in order to achieve pain-free, effective feeding.

- Emotional support and encouragement for the breastfeeding mother is also necessary while she overcomes any short-term problems, helping her to build her confidence in breastfeeding and her self-reliance, while also establishing her routine sources of support.

- Professional training should include (i) a sound knowledge of physical aspects of positioning and attachment; (ii) how to implement such knowledge, (iii) the opportunity to develop the skill to practice such knowledge with individual mothers and babies, and (iv) the ability to address all such matters sensitively, thereby empowering the mother and enhancing her self-esteem through her ability to feed her baby herself.

- Professionals should help women to understand that a pain-free, effective feeding technique is likely to be successful in overcoming most of the common problems of breastfeeding. They should be able to empower women to achieve this for themselves through the application of sound technical skills for positioning and attachment.

Further research **There is an urgent need for further research. A series of descriptive studies to identify the prevalence, types and natural history of the development of sore nipples and breasts is needed.** For example,

- how many women with sore nipples are not helped by correcting positioning techniques?
- how often are sore nipples associated with signs of infection, or problems in the baby such as tongue tie?
- do women develop breast pain in the absence of sore nipples, or are they always associated?
- how many women experience deep breast pain during and after feeds?

Such descriptive information is essential before developing trials of treatments.

5.2 Problems with milk flow

Breast engorgement

Despite the gradual move away from rigid feeding regimes to more flexible patterns of feeding, encouraging more frequent and effective milk flow, engorgement (fullness and oedema of the breast) and milk retention still cause tremendous discomfort and pain.

Prevention of engorgement

Studies summarised on pages 33–35 indicate that practices which encourage early breastfeeding, by a baby who is well positioned on the breast and whose spontaneous breastfeeding behaviour is not limited, will assist in the prevention of engorgement. There is some evidence that antenatal expression of colostrum may also have a role in the prevention of engorgement (see page 16).

One recent non-randomised comparison study compared two methods of feeding in an attempt to prevent engorgement (Evans et al 1995 [73]). Women in one group were encouraged to carry out prolonged feeding from one breast at each feed, although mothers were not prohibited from giving the baby the second breast if they and the baby wished. Women in the other group were asked to allow the baby to feed from both breasts equally. There was significantly less engorgement in the women in the group who carried out prolonged feeding from one breast at each feed.

Treatment of engorgement

Studies to examine the treatment of engorgement have examined three treatments: ultrasound, locally applied cabbage leaves, and proteolytic enzymes. Proteolytic enzymes are no longer available in the UK, but the evidence is reviewed here briefly, as they may still be in use in other countries.

ULTRASOUND

McLachlan et al (1991) [74] conducted a randomised double blind trial on ultrasound treatment for engorgement. They treated 197 breasts with either an ultrasound machine with the ultrasonic crystal in place or one where it had been removed. Neither the women nor the operator were aware which machine was active. The results showed no significant difference between the groups. Both treatments appeared to help, however, suggesting that the warmth, rest, massage and the practical information and support provided by the physiotherapists during treatment may have had a part to play.

CABBAGE LEAVES

The local application of cabbage leaves to engorged breasts is a practice which has evolved over the past two decades. It seems to have originated in 19th century France, but in recent years it has been used extensively in Australia, where it has become common practice. Its use has been evaluated in a randomised controlled trial of 120 women, in which the application of cabbage leaves at approximately

72 hours postpartum was compared to a control group. All women in both groups received 'routine care' which included daily 'breast exercises' (Nikodem et al 1993 [75]). No difference was found in engorgement, but significantly more women in the cabbage leaf group were still breastfeeding at 8 days and at 6 weeks after birth.

A further two small randomised trials have also examined the use of cabbage leaves for the relief of engorgement (Roberts 1995a [76] & 1995b [77]). One was a study in which 28 women were asked to use chilled cabbage leaves on one breast, and room temperature cabbage leaves on the other. No differences were found. The other, in which 34 women were asked to use chilled cabbage leaves on one breast and chilled gelpacks on the other breast, found a significant relief from pain with both treatments. Most mothers preferred the cabbage leaves.

PROTEOLYTIC ENZYMES

Two randomised controlled trials have examined the use of oral proteolytic enzymes (naturally-occurring plant enzymes) in the treatment of breast engorgement (Murata et al 1965 [78], Kee et al 1989 [79]). Both trials were double-blind, and women were allocated to either treatment of their engorgement with the proteolytic enzyme, or to receive a placebo. A total of 139 women were studied in the two trials. Both trials found a significant reduction in engorgement in the women who received the proteolytic enzyme, when compared with the women who received a placebo. No side effects were noted.

Discussion   There is a striking paucity of research examining this condition which is common, can be very painful, and has potentially hazardous consequences such as mastitis. There is evidence that some engorgement can be prevented by unlimited feeding by a baby who is well positioned at the breast, and by encouraging the woman to give a prolonged feed from one breast. No information is available to help identify the numbers and types of women who may become engorged even with good preventive care.

Evidence to guide treatment of the condition is also sparse. In summary, oral proteolytic enzymes (no longer available in the UK) and the local application of cabbage leaves may help. No other factors have been shown to work, but only ultrasound has been investigated in a randomised controlled trial.

PRACTICE IMPLICATIONS:

- Women who have just given birth should have access to practical, accurate support from appropriately trained professionals in order to ensure:
  - Pain-free, effective positioning of their baby at the breast
  - Flexible feeding patterns (i.e. frequent and of unrestricted length)
  Uninterrupted, effective feeding from the breast will ensure adequate milk removal and the avoidance of milk engorgement.

- In the absence of the baby, mechanical breast expression (hand or pump) may be necessary.

- The application of cold compresses or cabbage leaves (whether chilled or at room temperature) may result in some improvement or alleviation of symptoms, although this may be as a result of a placebo effect.

- Routine methods of relieving engorgement (improved feeding technique, hand expression, use of a breast pump, bathing or showering before a feed) may be equally effective if employed with expertise, enthusiasm and conviction by staff.

Further research   **There remain a number of important and unanswered questions:**
- What is the current incidence of engorgement among breastfeeding women in the UK, and what would the prevalence be if women were encouraged and supported in carrying out preventive measures?
- Does antenatal expression of colostrum help in the prevention of engorgement?
- Does the local application of cabbage leaves help, and if so, when and what are the best methods of using them?
- Is the evidence in favour of oral proteolytic enzymes strong enough to encourage further studies of their use?
- Would a regime such as that used in the ultrasound trial, including warmth, rest, breast massage and practical information and support, help women with engorgement?
- Would simple breast support, in the form of a well-fitting bra or breast binder, together with analgesia, help women with painful engorgement?
- Engorged breasts can become very swollen and hard, making it difficult for the baby to attach well. Are there techniques which would help women whose breasts are very swollen and painful to enable the baby to attach well to the breast?
- Would warm baths/showers and gentle expression help?

Many of the above questions could be effectively addressed in randomised controlled trials.

Mastitis

The term 'mastitis' may be used to refer to any inflammatory condition affecting the tissue of the breast, the presenting signs for which can range from simple focal inflammation, through development of a tender, hot, wedge-shaped segment of the breast, to involvement of the entire breast and advanced cellulitis. It can include the occurrence of systemic symptoms including pyrexia and those mimicking flu (shivers, rigor, fever, hot and cold flushes). It may, rarely, be related to the development of a breast abscess, which may in turn result in septicaemia.

Several distinct forms of localised or segmental breast inflammation may occur, all of which are likely to be referred to as 'mastitis', e.g. surface reddening to flushing of the entire breast surface, through to advanced cellulitis, with *peau d'orange* appearance. Such descriptions may deserve to be termed 'infective mastitis' to signify involvement of a pathogenic agent, although its presence is rarely verified by culture and sensitivity testing. In contrast, the presence of a discrete, localised, inflamed or tender area in one segment of the breast is more commonly caused either by blockage to a duct, or to obstruction of adequate milk flow, which can result in milk stasis leading to back-leakage of milk into the connective tissue surrounding the alveoli – such symptoms should probably be referred to as 'non-infective mastitis', although the absence of a pathogenic agent cannot be verified. Cases of mastitis may even be loosely referred to as an 'abscess' by health professionals, which would seem improbable when they resolve within 24 hours of initiating antibiotic therapy. Several authors use the term 'mastitis' rather indiscriminately, implying that all inflammatory conditions of the breast involve a pathogen, thus excluding the possibility that both a localised and a systemic immune response could be provoked simply by retrograde passage of unremoved milk either into the connective tissue of the breast or back into the blood stream, as first described by Gunther (1970).

Non-infective mastitis: Gunther described the condition of 'acute intramammary mastitis' as arising when milk pressure builds up within a group or cluster of alveoli to such an extent that it causes milk to leak between the mammary epithelial cells (paracellular pathway) back into the connective tissue surrounding the alveoli. Breast milk contains both anti-inflammatory agents and pyrogenic factors, so its presence in the connective tissue will provoke a localised immune response with inflammation and swelling; any such milk will eventually be re-absorbed. If this milk enters the circulation via the mammary capillaries the 'malaise' it can provoke 'is remarkably like that of the first stages of an incompatible blood transfusion' (Gunther, 1970).

A small number of descriptive studies have been carried out. Figures on the prevalence of the condition vary, probably as a result of both the definition of mastitis used and the method by which the population is sampled. Jonsson and Pulkkinen (1994) [80] questioned 664 women in outpatient clinics in Denmark, and found a reported prevalence of mastitis of 24%. Kaufmann and Foxman (1991) [81], however, in their retrospective cohort study of 966 lactating women, found only 2.9% of women reported an episode of mastitis. Riordan and Nichols (1990) [82] in their retrospective survey of mastitis in long-term breastfeeding women found that 33% of the 91 women surveyed had had at least one episode of mastitis.

Factors which have been associated with mastitis include fatigue, stress, and blocked ducts (Riordan and Nichols 1990 [82]). A survey of 100 women by Foxman et al (1994) [83], identified that 82% of women who developed mastitis had had pain in the breast or nipple in the week prior to the condition occurring.

Prevention of mastitis

The initial cause of non-infective mastitis appears to be milk stasis, and so the prevention of milk stasis is likely to be effective in preventing mastitis. Preventative measures should therefore include those summarised on pages 22–38. Practices which encourage early breastfeeding, by a baby who is well positioned on the breast and whose spontaneous breastfeeding behaviour is not limited, will assist in the prevention of mastitis.

Only one paper has been identified which examined directly the relationship between breast drainage and mastitis. Evans et al (1995) [73], in their non-randomised study, found no difference in the occurrence of mastitis in women who were asked to carry out a prolonged feed from one breast at each feed, compared with women who were asked to feed equally from both breasts at each feed. Inch and Fisher (1995) [84], however, found a strong negative association between the side on which mastitis occurred, and the side on which the mother preferred to hold her baby, suggesting an association between ineffective breast drainage and mastitis. Factors which prevent good drainage from the breast, or from part of the breast, should be avoided. These may include compression from restrictive clothing (e.g. a tight fitting bra), pressure from fingers, or from hands holding the breast tightly while feeding, or damage to the breast tissue resulting from trauma.

In cases of infective mastitis during breastfeeding, a pathogenic organism (commonly *Staphylococci spp*, but also *Streptococci*) invades the connective tissue of the breast, having gained entry through a fissure or lesion on the nipple surface. Infected milk, or retrograde movement of a skin commensal or pathogen from the baby's mouth into the milk ducts is unlikely to cause mastitis, although theoretically it might cause thickening of the milk predisposing to a plugged duct. However, the anti-infective agents present in breast milk probably act as the first line of defense against bacterial contamination of the milk.

Treatment of mastitis

Devereux (1969) [85] described the course of mastitis in 53 women, who had a total of 71 episodes of mastitis. He reported that when treatment (which included cold packs, continual nursing, analgesics and antibiotics) was delayed by more than 24 hours, women were likely to develop an abscess.

Thomsen et al (1984) [86] described three categories of mastitis classified on the basis of leucocyte counts and quantitative bacterial cultivation: *milk stasis* (defined as counts of $<10^6$ leukocytes and $<10^3$ bacteria per ml of milk), *non-infectious inflammation* ($>10^6$ leukocytes and $<10^3$ bacteria per ml of milk) and *infectious mastitis* ($>10^6$ leukocytes and $>10^3$ bacteria per ml of milk). Their results, from a randomised controlled trial, suggest that regular breast drainage improves the outcome in all groups, by shortening the episode, and reducing the severity of the outcome. *Non-infectious mastitis* did not appear to require antibiotics and no abscesses occurred when these were withheld, but giving antibiotics to women with *infectious mastitis* significantly reduced the numbers of women with abscesses.

Discussion   Mastitis is an important condition which can make the mother feel very unwell, and which can develop into an abscess, and even septicaemia. Its' prevention and treatment are very important. In spite of this, very little is known about the condition; there is no information, for example, on the prevalence of mastitis in the UK.

Prevention of the condition seems to be associated with good breast drainage. It is of interest that one paper has suggested that if the mother holds her baby more comfortably, perhaps the feeding is more effective from that side, thereby encouraging effective breast drainage (Inch and Fisher 1995).

Mastitis seems to be associated with the occurrence of blocked ducts. No research was found on the prevalence of, factors predisposing to, or treatment for, blocked ducts. Although some texts recommend regimes which include warm showers, gentle expression, and dietary modification, no tests or trials of such treatments have been reported. It is also possible that infective mastitis may be a result of nipple trauma which may allow entry of pathogens to the connective tissue, although no studies have examined this.

The results of the paper by Thomsen et al (1984) suggest that in deciding on appropriate treatment, it would be important to determine the type of mastitis which is presenting. The results of this paper suggest that women with milk stasis, non-infectious inflammation and infectious inflammation should all be encouraged to feed their baby regularly to promote drainage of the breast. Women with evidence of infectious inflammation should, in addition, have antibiotic treatment. Identification of such a group requires speedy access to leucocyte and bacterial counts, which is rare in this country. In the absence of this information, there is no evidence to suggest that women with mastitis should be given antibiotics as the first line of treatment. The evidence suggests that they should be encouraged to rest, helped to feed the baby frequently and effectively, and the course of the inflammation monitored. Should the condition not show signs of improvement within a few hours, antibiotic treatment should be considered (Note: The World Health Organization recommends a 24 hour delay before initiating antibiotic therapy; however, this recognises the difficulty that may be experienced in securing medical help in some parts of the world, so should perhaps be regarded as an upper limit).

PRACTICE IMPLICATIONS:

- Women need and should have ready access to practical, accurate support from appropriately trained professionals.

- Professionals require education concerning obstructive mastitis (resulting from milk retention or stasis) as a common cause of breast inflammation.

- Flexible feeding patterns with feeds which are frequent and of unrestricted length should be recommended.

- Prolonged effective feeding from the affected breast is needed to ensure effective milk removal and adequate drainage.

- Adjunctive use of mechanical breast expression may be of use in extreme cases.

- Where there are frank signs of bacterial infection (cellulitis, peau d'orange appearance of skin) antibiotics, which are effective against *Staphylococcus aureus* (flucloxacillin, augmentin), should be initiated without delay.

Further research   There remain a number of unanswered questions.
- **There is a need to determine both the incidence of mastitis in this country, and its prevalence at different stages of lactation.**
- Development of a simple differential diagnostic test to discriminate 'infective' mastitis from obstructive ('non-infective') mastitis in routine clinical practice.
- Based on accurate diagnosis of alternative forms of mastitis, the development of a range of appropriate treatments.
- Can mastitis be prevented by helping the mother to feed effectively from both breasts?
- Would the routine use of leucocyte and bacterial counts for women with mastitis be cost-effective as part of a treatment protocol?
- Are there other factors which cause mastitis? For example, illness, stress, exhaustion and blocked ducts are associated with its occurrence, and nipple trauma is a possible predisposing factor. What are the mechanisms which might cause this, and could this be prevented?
- Studies are needed to explore further the association noted with the mother's preferred holding side.
- An association has been noted between a family history of allergy and recurrent mastitis premenstrually (Minchin 1998). Is this the case? Is there a similar association with mastitis during breastfeeding? If so, what are the mechanisms, and can it be avoided?

5.3 Problems with milk supply

'Milk insufficiency'   The main reason given by women across the world for stopping breastfeeding before they planned to is that they have 'insufficient milk' (WHO 1981, Akre 1989, White et al 1992, Foster et al 1997). As outlined in the background to this paper, however, feeling that the milk supply is inadequate may be affected by social and psychological factors, as well as by physiological factors. In other words, the mother or her caregiver may believe that there is 'insufficient milk' to feed her baby, while there is in fact an adequate supply, or the potential to produce an adequate supply.

Women, and their caregivers, are likely to become concerned about the adequacy of the mothers' milk supply for a number of reasons, including the baby's crying, excessive feeding, changes in sleep pattern, a slower than expected weight gain, or weight loss. Infrequency or changes in the baby's stools may also contribute to this concern.

Care of women who feel they have 'insufficient milk' would be most effectively based on an accurate diagnosis of the problem (e.g. Woolridge 1995). In the current state of knowledge it is not possible in practice to differentiate between:
a. a physiological inability to produce enough milk
b. a transient and treatable reduction in milk supply resulting from a change in mother or baby's behaviour, or perhaps from a normal fluctuation in supply, or
c. a mother or caregiver's fear that the mother is not producing enough milk, for whatever reason

Very little research has been carried out on differentiating between these very different causes. Work in this field which is most likely to produce insights into the problem has been carried out in Australia (Daly et al 1993, 1996). These authors describe a method of measuring breast volume, the Computerised Breast Measurement System, which they have used to compare the change in breast volume before and after a feed. They found that the rate of milk synthesis was directly related to the degree the breast was emptied. The storage capacity of each breast varied from 81–606 ml. This research method offers new avenues for studying the relationship of maternal milk supply to infant demand for milk. It has been carried out on small numbers of women, however, and further work is needed, both to explore the development of this work for research, and possibly for use in clinical practice.

A perception of 'insufficient milk' may reflect an anxiety both with the amount of milk the baby is receiving, and the composition of that milk. Any diagnosis of problems with milk supply should include a consideration of the composition of milk the baby is receiving.

As a result of the lack of technology to guide practitioners working with women where milk insufficiency is suspected to be a problem, it is difficult for caregivers to make an accurate diagnosis. It is clear, however, that practitioners and women can be confident that a physiological inability to produce enough milk is greatly over-diagnosed. Such information as exists suggests that a physiological inability to produce enough milk may be found in no more than 1–5% of women (Neifert 1983). Among clinical referrals to a breastfeeding support service only 1.3% of women were found to have a pathophysiology of milk production (Woolridge 1995). A further 9.8% exhibited a proven impaired supply, although in over half of these it was 'acquired' (5.2%) rather than 'intrinsic' (4.8%). The vast majority of all referrals to the clinic for breast milk insufficiency (55% of the 66%, i.e. 83%) were transient and correctable.

Causes of 'insufficient milk'

Iatrogenic

Given the information described in all the preceding sections of this paper, it is likely that although many women feel they have 'insufficient milk', it may in part be an iatrogenic problem, resulting from inappropriate restrictions on feeding, unresolved positioning problems, and a lack of accurate, consistent advice and support (Woolridge 1995).

Social and psychological factors

The social and psychological context of breastfeeding (pages 9–11) can make it very difficult for women to have confidence in the fact that they have a milk supply which is more than adequate to feed their baby. In a culture where so many women stop feeding as a result of problems, where conflicting advice is given by caregivers, and where family support may be lacking, women questioning whether or not they can sustain their own baby without help is an inevitable consequence.

Physical factors

Physical problems may result in an inability to produce milk. A small number of studies have examined such factors, including blood loss at birth, and drugs which may influence milk supply.

BLOOD LOSS

Two studies have examined anaemia and haemorrhage, and the possible effect on milk production (Willis and Livingstone 1995 [87], Henly et al 1995 [88]). Willis and Livingstone studied ten women who had a postpartum haemorrhage (reported blood loss ranged from 500 to 1500 mls) and whose babies were referred to a breastfeeding clinic with a history of failure to thrive. On the basis of these case studies, they suggest that a postpartum haemorrhage can produce a transient hypotensive insult and a resultant temporary pituitary ischaemia which inhibits the hormonal triggering of lactogenesis by prolactin.

Henly et al (1995) [88] followed up 630 women who started to breastfeed in their study of anaemia and 'insufficient milk'. Twenty two percent of these women (137) had a postpartum haemoglobin level of less than 10g/dl, of which almost 20% of women with anaemia reported 'insufficient milk syndrome'; this was significantly greater than the 11% of those who were not anaemic.

- Professionals should be aware of the small number of pathophysiological causes of true milk insufficiency

- They should also be aware that the majority of cases of reported, perceived or transient 'insufficiency' can be simply corrected by applying sound technical skills to ensure pain-free, effective feeding and by providing support and reassurance for the mother.

- Accordingly, basic knowledge and skills are essential to empower mothers to practice sound breastfeeding technique, and to manage breastfeeds optimally in order to minimise the occurrence of perceived insufficiency.

- Community health professionals also need to know how to interpret measurements of the baby's weight appropriately, in order to determine when poor/inadequate growth requires specialist evaluation of breastfeeding.

- Special counselling skills are required to help mothers cope with a crying, unsettled baby, and how to recognise other potential causes of a baby's distress or discomfort.

- There is a need, perhaps, to improve the ability of community health professionals to address basic parenting skills with parents, and to educate them accordingly.

- Education of the general public is needed to dispel the myth that underfeeding is the main (and only) cause of distressed behaviour in babies, and to ensure that women are not subjected to social pressures to comply with unrealistic expectations about breastfeeding.

Further research   There is a need to reach a medical consensus as to the limited set of patho-physiological conditions which contraindicate the success of lactation. There is a further need to ascertain which clinical conditions can cause transient impairment of milk output, and of the possible therapeutic options which are available to overcome such problems. Only when the tiny proportion of medical conditions have been elucidated, can attention turn to addressing non-organic causes of perceived milk insufficiency.

The problem of 'insufficient milk' (whether reported or substantiated) deserves formal recognition as clinical entity, capable of being verified or not by appropriate investigations. The research needed to achieve this will involve clinicians and practitioners in the field, and basic biomedical researchers (physiologists & biochemists). Given that breastfeeding is more likely to fail for socio-cultural reasons than for biological ones, there is an equal need to address the socio-cultural basis of 'milk insufficiency'. Such work must involve wide-ranging, multi-disciplinary research engaging sociologists and anthropologists, as well as consumers.

Prevention of 'insufficient milk'

Identifying women likely to develop 'milk insufficiency' There is little evidence to assist in the identification of women who may develop milk insufficiency, and who may benefit especially from preventive measures. Neifert et al (1990) [89], in their descriptive study of 319 women, found that women with insufficient lactation were more likely to report minimal, or absent, prenatal breast enlargement, and minimal postnatal breast engorgement. Women with peri-areolar breast incisions (arising from surgical breast augmentation or reduction mammoplasty) were nearly 5 times more likely to have lactation insufficiency. A descriptive study of 47 women (Houston et al 1983b [90]) found that women with low milk production in the first 6 days after birth were more likely to stop breastfeeding at six weeks.

The studies summarised above on pages 22–38 indicate that practices which encourage early breastfeeding, by a baby who is well positioned at the breast and whose spontaneous feeding behaviour is not limited, will increase the duration of breastfeeding and reduce the numbers of women stopping as a result of 'insufficient milk'. In addition to this, there is a strong body of evidence to indicate that women who receive support and appropriate advice are more likely to continue to breastfeed and less likely to discontinue feeding as a result of 'insufficient milk'.

Fluids and diet The practice of encouraging women to drink more fluids to prevent 'insufficient milk' and to promote a good milk supply has been examined in two small studies (Morse et al 1992 [91], Dearlove and Dearlove 1981[92]). These studies found no evidence that increasing maternal fluid intake affected either the prolactin levels or the breast milk supply.

PRACTICE IMPLICATIONS:

- Continued general and specific education on how breastfeeding works (in particular, milk supply and demand) is needed for both mothers and professionals alike.

- 'Effective delivery of the milk manufactured' is the key to ensuring the baby is settled after feeding; this is dependent upon implementation of sound physiological principles regarding positioning and attachment. Professionals need to be aware of other causes of irritability and distress in newborn.

- There is no evidence that dietary modification or manipulating fluid intake is of therapeutic benefit.

Further research Women who are self-confident and have an effective social support network appear to be relatively resilient to concerns about their milk supply. Women are more likely to be at risk, however, if they lack effective practical or social support (e.g. absence of a partner); if they are disadvantaged by social circumstances (e.g. overcrowded housing, in receipt of social financial benefits); if their social network only comprises inappropriate role models for breastfeeding (e.g. their mother bottle-fed); or if their personality is such that they have low self-esteem or an intrinsic lack of self-confidence. Identification of such 'at-risk' women should mean that appropriate care can be more effectively targeted, and be offered with greater sensitivity to the needs of such women. Such information is likely to come from a combination of quantitative and ethnographic research (for example, see Victora et al 1997).

Treatment of 'insufficient milk'

Given the evidence described above and on pages 22–38, there are good grounds for assuming that unrestricted breastfeeding by an infant who is well positioned at the breast, and the receipt of support, encouragement and sound advice, may help those women who are experiencing either a transient and treatable reduction in milk supply, or a culturally induced fear of 'insufficient milk'. It may also be the case that such support and encouragement may maximise milk production in women with physiological problems in producing enough milk.

Only one study has been identified of women with 'lactation failure' who were provided with such supportive measures. Mathur et al (1992) [93] report their experiences of working with 75 women with partial or complete 'lactation failure'. Complete lactation failure was defined as 'total absence of milk flow or secretion of only a few drops of milk following regular suckling for a period of at least 7 days'. Partial lactation failure was defined as 'mothers spontaneously complained of inadequate milk flow and the infants required artificial milk feeding'. Relactation was defined as 'resumption of breastfeeding following cessation or significant decrease in milk production'. All women were encouraged to relactate. Mothers were provided with adequate rest, nutrition and psychological support. Frequent and prolonged feeding by the baby in the proper position, and the immediate cessation of pacifiers and bottles, was advised. If additional feeding was required, it was given only after breastfeeding was attempted. If lactation was not established, metoclopramide 10mg was given 8 hourly for 10 days; no figures are given for the number of women who had drug treatment. If this regime did not succeed, a nursing supplementer (a fine, long tube attached to the mother's breast and nipple through which the baby can suck milk from a cup or bottle while at the breast) was used. Following the use of this regime, 49 (70%) of women with partial lactation failure successfully relactated. Three of the four women with complete lactation failure were also successful. The authors attribute the cause of the breastfeeding problems in these women to the fact that 'most of the women did not receive appropriate support for breastfeeding'. This paper suggests that over 70% of women with serious breastfeeding problems related to milk supply can have a successful outcome.

These results are supported by a description of the outcomes for women referred to a breastfeeding clinic in Bristol (Woolridge 1995). Seven hundred and five women received consultations over a two and a half year period, four hundred and sixty five of whom presented with 'low milk output'. Of these, 85% of the cases were resolved by simple advice and support. Fewer than 2% were attributed to pathophysiological failure of milk production

Hillervik-Lindquist (1991) [94], in her descriptive study of providing support to women with 'transient lactation crises' reported that continuous support and prompt access to help could prevent cessation of breastfeeding due to perceived breast milk insufficiency. This study demonstrated that although 28 mothers out of 51 experienced transient lactation crisis, it was possible to increase the breast-feeding rate with mothers having access to continuous support and prompt access to help save acute lactational problems.

Drug treatment Drugs used in an effort to promote lactation include dopamine antagonists and thyrotrophin releasing hormone (TRH), which cause an increase in prolactin levels; and syntocinon (synthetic oxytocin), which elicits the let-down reflex. One small trial was identified which examined the use of human growth hormone, while two small studies, one descriptive and one randomised controlled trial, examined the effect of traditional herbal preparations on milk supply.

Dopamine antagonists examined include metoclopramide, sulpiride, domperidone and chlorpromazine. Side effects of metoclopramide and sulpiride are reported to include sedation, dystonia, raised blood pressure and a Parkinson-like syndrome following prolonged use (Martindale 1982). Babies may experience extrapyramidal dystonia and tardive dyskinesia (Silb and Glass 1978). Domperidone is claimed not to cross the blood-brain barrier, so is less likely to provoke extrapyramidal side effects (Reyntjens et al 1978).

Details of the studies, all of which are small, are given in the tables. Summary results only will be given here.

METOCLOPRAMIDE

Six studies (Guzman et al 1979 [95], Lewis et al 1980 [96], Kauppila et al 1981a [97],1981b [98] & 1988 [99], and de Gezelle et al 1983 [100]) were identified.

A small study of 20 women post-caesarean section (Lewis et al 1980 [96]) found no difference in the success at establishing lactation among treated and untreated women. Mothers' serum prolactin levels were measured in the other five studies and in all metoclopramide was found to result in increased basal pro-lactin levels. Milk yield, in contrast, was more variable in response. In one study of women who wanted to improve milk production [99] an increase in milk output was only found after 3 weeks of treatment (at a dose of 30mg/day). Detectable changes were more prompt in two studies both of women without problems [100] and of those with a previous history of poor lactation [95]. In two remaining studies of women reporting 'insufficient lactation', milk output was only measured after 2 or 3 weeks of treatment had elapsed [97, 98]. It was also the case in the latter two studies, however, that breast milk output returned swiftly to pre-treatment levels when metoclopramide was withdrawn [98] or replaced by a placebo [97]. In one case [98] the levels of serum prolactin even fell below pre-treatment levels, suggesting a possible 'rebound' response to withdrawal of metoclopramide.

One further study of 23 women, who were mechanically expressing their milk by electric pump for their premature baby (Ehrenkranz & Ackerman 1986), noted both an increase in milk yield (in all 17 women for whom it was measured) and an increase in basal serum prolactin (in all 6 women measured) one week after initiating metoclopramide therapy. Although the results of this study may seem encouraging, no placebo control group was used, and the fact that the women were expressing their milk gave them feedback as to the efficacy of treatment.

Mathur (1992) [93] described the use of metoclopramide for women with lactation failure, but as a last resort, after trying support, rest, nutrition, encouragement, positioning and other supportive measures. No data were given on the numbers of women who needed metoclopramide, but a 70–75% rate of successful relactation was described.

SULPIRIDE

Four studies (Aono et al 1979 [101] & 1982 [102], and Ylikorkala et al 1984a [103] & 1984b [104]) showed that, in women with 'inadequate lactation', sulpiride increases basal serum prolactin and daily milk yield. The increases in milk yield, however, were not accompanied by a decrease in the numbers of women discontinuing breastfeeding, so may not prove to be of practical significance. Side effects from drug use were reported.

DOMPERIDONE

Petraglia et al (1985 [105]) and Hofmeyr (1985 [106]) examined the use of oral domperidone in two very small studies. Petraglia et al (1985) examined 32 women with lactation problems, and found minimal serum prolactin increases, and an increased milk yield on the 10th day of treatment. Hofmeyr (1985) studied 10 women whose infants were temporarily unable to take breast milk, and found an increase in serum prolactin. They did not measure milk yield.

TRH

Ylikorkala et al (1980 [107]), Peters et al (1991 [108]) and Zarate et al (1976 [109a & 109b]) have examined the use of TRH. Again, the studies were small, but all found an increase in basal serum prolactin. Only Peters et al (1991) noted an increase in milk yield in the seven women in their TRH group, but their study examined women with low milk yield, in contrast to that of Zarate (1976), which examined women after birth, with normal lactation.

OXYTOCIN

The use of oxytocin was examined by Friedman and Sachtleben (1961), Huntingford (1961), Luhman (1963) and Ylikorkala et al (1984b [104] in combination with sulpiride). Buccal and nasal preparations were used, which are no longer available in this country. There is no convincing evidence that this drug is effective, but the trials are small.

HUMAN GROWTH HORMONE

One randomised controlled trial of 16 women (Milsom et al 1992 [110]) has examined the use of human growth hormone in healthy breastfeeding women, between 8-18 weeks after birth. Their results indicated an increase in milk volume after seven days of treatment; although statistically significant, the increase in milk volume (37 mls in 24 hours) is unlikely to be clinically significant at this age.

HERBAL PREPARATIONS

One small descriptive study examined the use of a herbal extract of *Leptadenia reticulata* and *Breynia patens* ('Leptaden') (Gokhale 1965 [111]). Twenty five women with a history of 'lactation failure' were given the drug, but there was no evidence that its use was effective. A randomised controlled trial, involving 64 women, of a root extract of *Asparagus racemosus* ('Shatavari') (Sharma et al 1996 [112]) was unable to show any impact on prolactin levels, infant weight gain or use of supplemental fluids.

To summarise the results of studies on drugs to increase milk supply, there is little evidence that the use of anti-dopamine drugs (excepting sulpiride) will produce a reliable increase in milk output, particularly for mothers with established low milk output, although maternal serum prolactin levels were elevated reliably by their use. In light of their potential side effects, and the possibility that withdrawal may provoke a rapid reversal of any therapeutic benefit, they should not be used in routine practice (nor are they licensed for such use in the UK). Evidence that TRH is effective is also equivocal. Further studies are needed to establish the relationship between elevated serum prolactin levels and the presence/absence of changes in milk output, both for women with reduced lactation and for women with potentially normal lactation who are temporarily unable to feed their babies. There is no evidence to support the use of oxytocin (which is no longer available in the UK), human growth hormone, or herbal preparations.

Discussion   Mothers who fear that their babies are not receiving enough milk are usually highly anxious and in need of support and good care. It is astonishing that there remains such a lack of good evidence to inform women and practitioners, and to guide practice, in relation to the leading cause of breastfeeding failure worldwide. It is still not possible in practice to distinguish between women who have a physiological cause underlying their inability to satisfy their baby, and those whose milk supply is affected by social or psychological factors; research in this field is only in early stages of development. Routine measures to prevent 'insufficient milk' are fairly well established, however, and ways of putting them into practice should be more critically examined.

The descriptive study by Mathur et al (1992) in India is the only example of a study which investigates a regime of care which combines physical and psychosocial factors. The care they offered women, which appeared to be very successful, suggest that it is possible to successfully treat a very high proportion of women with 'insufficient milk' – even those identified as having 'total lactation failure'.

In all of the plethora of studies examining drug treatment for this condition, only Mathur et al (1992) examined the use of a drug in combination with other supportive measures. The other striking aspect of these studies is the fact that all are small, and that the crucial questions of clinical relevance, such as milk yield, duration of breastfeeding, and weight gain in the baby, have not been well addressed. In addition, there are obvious distinctions to be drawn between women with reduced lactation for physical and social/emotional reasons, and women with potentially normal lactation who cannot feed their babies and need support to continue under difficult circumstances. No studies have examined this essential question.

PRACTICE IMPLICATIONS:

- Professionals must be knowledgeable about the physical mechanics of milk removal, how to employ this knowledge to maximise the quantity of milk removed from the breast (and hence its energy content), and how the baby exercises appetite control in order to self-regulate calorie or fat intake.

- Knowledge and skills are required to detect and tackle alternative causes of distressed behaviour in infants, e.g. colic.

- Women who are noted to have a heavy blood loss at birth, or to be anaemic, should receive additional attention postnatally to ensure that their milk supply is not adversely affected.

- Specialist outpatient facilities are required to evaluate cases of poor or inadequate growth in the breastfed infant to determine whether underfeeding is the cause (as opposed to an intrinsic organic problem in the infant).

Further research   There remain many unanswered questions which deserve to be addressed.

- Work is needed to distinguish the different types of 'milk insufficiency', and to differentiate those which have a true pathophysiological basis from those which are non-organic in origin (i.e. acquired, iatrogenic or behaviourally-induced).
- Do women who are anaemic, or who have a heavy blood loss at birth, have subsequent problems with milk production? If so, are there any interventions which alleviate such problems?
- A programme of supportive care (such as that described by Mathur et al, 1992) should be tested in a randomised controlled trial. Supportive care could be targeted at specific groups such as
    (i) women with 'insufficient milk',
    (ii) women with babies in neonatal units,
    (iii) women 'at risk' of discontinuation of breastfeeding (e.g. socio-economically disadvantaged).
- Would dopamine antagonists (e.g. domperidone, metoclopramide) enhance lactation for:
    (i) women in the community who are lacking effective sources of support,
    (ii) women who also receive supportive care, and
    (iii) women separated from their babies, who must sustain their lactation by breast expression?
- Treatments which are often advised for 'insufficient milk', including
    (i) prolonged feeding from one breast at each feed,
    (ii) breast massage,
    (iii) supplementing babies who show slow weight gain.
    These could be evaluated by randomised controlled trials.
- Evaluate effective ways of:
    (i) restoring lost confidence, and
    (ii) overcoming crises of confidence (peer support schemes)
- Evaluation of the predictive ability of clinical investigations (milk volume measurement, assessment of milk fat content, hormone levels, ultrasound examination of the breast and/or baby's mouth) and of their role during follow-up in cases of perceived or substantiated breast milk insufficiency.
- Can self-help guides targeted at women experiencing 'perceived milk insufficiency' be as effective as personal contact and support?

A coordinated programme of work is needed to address appropriately the interrelated physical, psychological, professional, social and cultural issues.

6 | Baby-related problems

Although it is difficult to separate the mother and baby when considering breast-feeding, there are some areas where (a) the method of feeding may be associated with problems in the baby (for example, jaundice, and 'colic' or inconsolable crying), or (b) the baby's condition makes breastfeeding difficult (for example, Down's syndrome, cleft lip and palate, and tongue tie).

One further issue not reviewed in this paper, but which is essential for mothers of babies with feeding difficulties, is the best means of initiating and maintaining a good milk supply by breast expression. Expression of breast milk has been reviewed recently (Drane et al 1994) and the types of pump available have been described by others (Walker & Auerbach 1993).

This section will summarise the research evidence related to baby-related problems. The care of premature and sick babies was outside the scope of this review.

6.1 Hypoglycaemia

One of the more controversial areas in the care of the normal, term breastfed baby is the prevention, detection and management of hypoglycaemia. The literature relating to this issue is extensive and is the subject of a comprehensive review prepared for the World Health Organization (Williams 1997). We have not reviewed this field, therefore, but have chosen instead to highlight selected conclusions drawn, or extrapolated, from Williams' review, on which the guidelines published by the National Childbirth Trust (NCT) (1997) were subsequently based:

Routine management of asymptomatic babies

There is no necessity to test *normal, healthy term* infants routinely for low blood sugar, so long as they show appropriate vital signs and are asymptomatic. Healthy term babies do not develop clinical signs of hypoglycaemia simply as a result of underfeeding. Furthermore, there is no convincing evidence that hypoglycaemia detected in such infants has persisting or irreversible clinical consequences.

Exclusive, unrestricted breastfeeding, initiated at the earliest opportunity after birth, should satisfy the baby's entire liquid and nutrient needs. Awareness should be maintained, however, of the potential for artificial interventions during labour and birth (pharmacological analgesia for example) or unnatural practices (such as enforced separation of the mother from her infant resulting in a drop in the baby's body temperature) to adversely affect the baby's tendency and ability to feed, or his/her glucose requirements. Close physical contact, skin-to-skin where possible, should be maintained between the mother and her newborn to minimise heat loss by the baby which might lead to increased glucose needs – both may be covered if the mother feels cold. A short-lived decline in blood glucose level in the first 24 hours after birth is a normal physiological adaptation to extra-uterine life by the newborn.

Management of the baby who doesn't wake to feed

Babies who cannot be regarded as normal, healthy term infants may include those who will not feed or do not wake to be fed. It is recommended that certain simple procedures be followed to exclude an abnormality or underlying illness, which include physical observation and clinical examination in preference to routine blood sugar testing; simply giving artificial formula to a baby detected as 'hypoglycaemic' on blood glucose testing might delay the investigation of an incipient condition or disease.

In consequence, if there are no signs of illness but the feeding is still regarded as 'abnormal', a cycle of "FEED-CHECK-REVIEW" is recommended as the more appropriate course of action than blood sugar testing and supplementary feeding alone (NCT 1997). This would include attempts to rouse the baby and offer the breast, the offering of expressed breast milk by cup if appropriate, examination of the baby's physical signs, followed by review of the overall situation. Under all circumstances, the mother's (parents') informed consent should be secured prior to giving a supplementary feed. It is urged that the atopic history of both parents be ascertained as part of this process.

'Symptomatic' hypoglycaemia

In contrast, babies who show signs of hypoglycaemia (abnormalities of tone or conscious level), confirmed by laboratory blood sugar testing, should be investigated for the possible cause of their hypoglycaemia, and intra-venous glucose should be started immediately to correct it. Symptomatic hypoglycaemia may be of intrinsic organic origin, such as a systemic infection or an inborn error of metabolism, so it should not be assumed that infants who are found to be hypoglycaemic simply need to be fed. Advising that the baby be fed and re-tested after an interval is likely to delay the investigation, detection and delivery of appropriate treatment for the true cause.

A fuller list of pathological conditions associated with abnormal glucose homeostasis is provided by Williams (1997).

Babies at risk of hypoglycaemia

Objective criteria can be set down for infants who might be considered at risk of hypoglycaemia. These are: preterm babies, babies who are small for gestational age, babies who are cold, ill or have an infection, or a baby born to a diabetic mother. These babies should be monitored according to local policy and their mothers offered help with breastfeeding. If additional fluids are needed babies should be offered expressed breast milk or dextrose to raise their blood glucose. With the exception of babies born to diabetic mothers, babies who are simply large-for-dates are not at risk.

Routine management

Wherever possible, non-intrusive interventions, such as efforts to rouse the baby, offering expressed colostrum or breastmilk by syringe, spoon or cup, are preferable to routine blood sugar testing or of supplementing babies with formula by bottle. Policies should be formulated which place reliance on clinical assessment and observation of the baby and on routine checks, together with documentation of breastfeeds, including their quality.

Clinically relevant levels

There is an absence of data concerning what constitutes a clinically relevant level for defining hypoglycaemia in the normal term infant; that is, a level likely to lead to irreversible neurological impairment. A multi-centre study of at-risk preterm infants has shown neurological impairment from hypoglycaemia (plasma glucose <2.6 mmols) lasting more than 72 hours. It would be inappropriate, however, to apply such a measure to the normal term infant.

Normal, healthy term infants are capable of utilising other sources of energy to supply the brain, such as lactate and ketone bodies and are not solely reliant on glucose in the blood stream (Hawdon et al 1992). Preterm infants are less able to mobilise ketone bodies as a source of energy, and in one study (Koh et al, 1988) which suggested impaired neurological function (e.g. prolonged latency of auditory evoked potentials) the babies were hypoketonaemic as well as hypoglycaemic.

Mechanism of testing

The routine testing of blood sugar levels using glucose reagent strips should be discontinued as they are of insufficient accuracy and sensitivity for this task (as previously recommended by Cornblath et al, 1990). Laboratory tests should be used or measurements made using a glucose electrode.

Several practice implications, based on these conclusions, are proposed below:

PRACTICE IMPLICATIONS:

- Early initiation of breastfeeding should be encouraged.

- Newly delivered mothers will need practical, accurate support from appropriately trained professionals at the first and subsequent feeds.

- Flexible feeding patterns, comprising frequent feeds of unrestricted length, should be encouraged.

- There should be greater acceptance by health professionals that long interfeed intervals during the early days after birth can be normal in the healthy, term newborn.

- It is essential to differentiate the healthy term newborn from the 'at-risk' infant; the principles of breastfeeding management set out above apply to the healthy term newborn.

- In order to differentiate the normal, healthy term infant from the 'at-risk' infant it may be prudent to clinically assess and document the quality of the first feeds at the breast.

- Maternity units should develop policy guidelines for identifying infants at risk of hypoglycaemia (refer to Williams, 1997), and both monitor its implementation and audit relevant outcomes.

- There needs to be greater understanding among professionals that underfeeding should not be regarded as the sole or primary cause of detectable hypoglycaemia. In cases of persistent or symptomatic hypoglycaemia the infant should be investigated for an underlying condition, such as neonatal infection.

- Paediatric consensus is needed over the clinical definition of hypoglycaemia in 'at-risk' infants, thereby defining which infants should be formally screened.

- Appropriate methods should be used for measuring blood glucose level (e.g. laboratory glucose electrode) where a paediatric decision has been made that an 'at-risk' baby should be monitored.

- Inappropriate methods for measuring blood glucose level (e.g. glucose oxidase reagent strips) should be abandoned.

- A cycle of "FEED-CHECK-REVIEW" is recommended for the baby who has slept for a period which either the mother or staff feel is unacceptable. Efforts should be made to rouse the baby and offer the breast as the first option; alternatively, the baby can be offered expressed breast milk by cup, spoon, syringe or tube as appropriate.

6.2 Jaundice

Jaundice is a manifestation of raised serum bilirubin levels in the baby. In the normal, term newborn, jaundice can be defined as either early-onset or 'physiological' jaundice, or late-onset, sometimes referred to as 'breastmilk jaundice'. Early-onset jaundice is common, while late-onset jaundice has been estimated to affect a very small percentage of babies. Auerbach and Gartner (1987) provide a thorough review of these conditions. Prolonged jaundice can indicate an incipient liver disorder and so needs to be discriminated from unresolved physiological jaundice or breast-milk jaundice.

The ramifications from a diagnosis of jaundice can either be beneficial or harmful. Invariably it results in active intervention (e.g. prescribing phototherapy, scheduled feeds, taking regular blood samples to measure bilirubin levels) which often involve separation of the mother from her baby, efforts to dictate the timing of breastfeeds, and giving additional feeds of formula or water. In some cases, perhaps especially cases of long-term, late-onset jaundice which may persist for several weeks, mothers may be advised to take the baby off the breast altogether.

The small number of studies identified investigated early-onset jaundice. No studies of late-onset jaundice were identified.

Johnson et al (1985) [48] found a negative association between weight loss on the third day, and serum bilirubin levels. Breastfed babies had the highest serum bilirubin levels. Adams et al (1985) [113] similarly found a higher incidence of hyperbilirubinaemia in breastfed babies, in their descriptive study of 233 healthy term babies.

Prevention of jaundice

Studies which investigated the effect of routine practices such as supplementation on the occurrence of jaundice were described above, on pages 38–41. In summary, giving routine additional fluids, or feeding by schedule every three hours instead of every four, made no difference to the numbers of babies with raised serum bilirubin levels.

Restricting the baby's spontaneous feeding behaviour by schedule feeding, whether every three or four hours may, however, result in increased levels of jaundice. One study indicated that the more feeds the baby takes, the less likely it is that jaundice will develop. In de Carvalho et al's (1982) [114] descriptive study of 55 mother-infant pairs, an association was found between frequency of feeding and serum bilirubin concentrations. Babies who had more than 8 feeds in 24 hours during the first three days had significantly lower levels than those who fed fewer than 8 times.

Treatment of jaundice

Three studies of treatment for babies with jaundice were identified.

Martinez et al (1993) [46] studied 125 healthy, term babies who had raised serum bilirubin levels. They were randomised to one of four groups: continue breastfeeding and observe; discontinue breastfeeding, and give formula; discontinue breastfeeding, give formula and phototherapy; and continue breastfeeding, and give phototherapy. The results presented are limited, and give no information on the continuation of breastfeeding. Bilirubin levels fell fastest in the groups receiving phototherapy. Of babies in the group who were asked to continue breastfeeding without intervention, only 24% had a bilirubin level of over 342 micromoles/litre. The highest recorded bilirubin level was 393 micro-moles/litre. No babies required exchange transfusion, and all babies remained clinically well.

One non-randomised prospective study (de Carvalho et al 1981 [47]) compared the use of water supplementation with no supplementation in term, healthy babies with physiological jaundice. There was no significant difference between the groups in serum bilirubin levels, or in the number of babies requiring phototherapy.

Elander and Lindberg (1986) [115] carried out a small, non-randomised study in which mothers of babies with hyperbilirubinaemia were allocated to two groups – one in which babies were sent to the neonatal unit for phototherapy as usual – mothers were therefore separated from their babies; and one group in which mothers and babies were cared for together in a single room, where babies also received phototherapy. At 12 weeks, significantly more women from the non-separated group were still breastfeeding. Women reported that they much preferred to be with their babies.

Discussion   There is a surprising lack of well-conducted research about this condition, which is very common, and which often results in serious disruption of breastfeeding and of the relationship between the mother and her baby. Such research as exists suggests that this condition may in part be iatrogenic, resulting from restrictions on feeding and contact between mother and baby, and giving additional fluids. Evidence suggests that no limitations should be imposed on normal, spontaneous breastfeeding behaviour in an effort to avoid physiological jaundice. Physiological jaundice may best be prevented by encouraging frequent, uninterrupted breastfeeding. For example, the laxative effect of colostrum in the first 48 hours is likely to speed up the excretion of meconium and prevent the reabsorption of bile pigments. Additional fluids, or the restriction of breastfeeding, may interfere with this mechanism.

When such jaundice occurs, treatment ought to be in proportion to the problem. For example, in the absence of complicating factors such as infection or prematurity, it is highly unlikely that physiological jaundice will reach levels which requires major intervention. If babies do require phototherapy, care should be taken to avoid disrupting the relationship between mother and baby, and to support breastfeeding.

No studies were identified which examined the treatment of late-onset, or 'breastmilk' jaundice. Clinical experience recommends that a short suspension of breastfeeding (24–36hr at the most) permits bilirubin levels to fall to a level at which they are manageable within the context of continued breastfeeding (Auerbach & Gartner 1987)

PRACTICE IMPLICATIONS:

- Early feeding should be encouraged (in view of the laxative effect of colostrum) to reduce the impact of physiological jaundice.

- There is no benefit from giving supplementary water, so this practice should be discontinued. There are also other more appropriate fluids than water to be given to prevent dehydration during phototherapy; these include expressed breast milk.

- Flexible feeding patterns – frequent feeds of unrestricted length – should be encouraged (maximising fat/calorie intake facilitates the breakdown of bilirubin).

- Mothers should have access to practical accurate support from appropriately trained professionals.

- Do not separate mothers and babies when phototherapy is needed, so that the mother may respond as soon as her baby shows signs of wanting to be fed.

Further research
- A large study in an environment where breastfeeding is well managed would help to identify the numbers of babies who develop serious levels of jaundice even when breastfeeding is unrestricted and no unnecessary interventions are carried out.
- Work is needed to identify the prevalence of and best management for late-onset jaundice

6.3 Crying and 'colic'

A mother's anxiety about her baby's crying may often manifest itself in anxiety about breastfeeding. This may result in her feeling that she has 'insufficient milk', or that her milk is abnormal in some way, such as 'too weak' or 'too rich'. She may also worry that her baby has 'colic'. This distressing condition manifests as a combination of behaviours from inconsolable crying, to high-pitched wailing or screaming. This signals to the mother that her baby is in pain or distress, with the baby's tendency to draw up his/her knees being regarded by some as indicating abdominal cramps (Riordan & Auerbach 1993) and by others to be of little significance (Taubman 1990). It can be difficult for mothers and caregivers to distinguish colic from other signs of distress in the baby, and like 'insufficient milk', colic is likely to be overdiagnosed.

Whether or not crying is seen as a problem will depend on the response of the immediate family. A baby who cries for two hours a day may be seen as quite normal by one family, and as having a major problem by another family. Responses may be modulated by whether or not the baby exhibits any other symptoms such as slow weight gain, whether or not the mother has had difficult experiences in the past, whether or not she is well supported by family, friends and caregivers, and whether or not she knows and understands the normal range of baby behaviour. There is a large element of subjectivity in people's responses, resulting in this being a very difficult area to study and to understand.

Studies which examine ways of preventing or treating crying or colic in breastfed babies are rare, however. Studies which examined allergies and food intolerance, although having an important contribution to knowledge in this area, were outside the scope of this review.

One non-randomised study examined the effect of feeding technique on colic in breastfed babies (Evans et al 1995 [73]). A total of 302 women were allocated to two groups. One group were encouraged to carry out prolonged feeding from one breast, using the second breast only if the baby was still hungry. Women in the other group were asked to feed from both breasts equally at each feed. Among other outcomes, women were asked at six months after birth if their babies suffered from colic (defined as episodes of inconsolable crying, thought to be due to abdominal pain and requiring medication or medical advice). Of the women who were asked to carry out prolonged feeding on one breast, 12% reported such colic, compared with 23% asked to feed from both breasts (p<0.02).

The study of Evans et al (1995) was devised to test the hypothesis proposed by Woolridge and Fisher (1988). Based on clinical studies and a knowledge of the changes in breast milk composition, this hypothesis proposed that babies may suffer colic and symptoms of lactose malabsorption (failure to thrive, colic and irritability, and watery diarrhoea) as a result of incorrect feed management. The common practice at that time of asking women to feed equally from both breasts, by taking the baby off the first breast after a maximum of 10 minutes and putting him or her on the second breast, may result in some babies receiving large amounts of low-fat foremilk, and very little high-fat hindmilk. The authors concluded that the baby should be permitted to finish the first breast first, by letting the baby come off spontaneously, then be offered the second breast to take if he/she wishes. In this way the baby would be enabled to regulate his/her own intake to secure a natural balance of foremilk and hindmilk.

One other study was identified which tested this hypothesis. Righard et al (1993 [116]) randomised 80 mothers on a maternity ward, who were already following a two-breast per feed pattern as part of standard care, to either a one- or two-breast per feed pattern. For mothers changing their pattern of feeding, compliance was poor, with 52% not adhering to protocol. Nonetheless, among those who established the new pattern, there were no differences in maternal satisfaction, mood or confidence at one month. Similarly, there were no significant differences in the frequency of feeding, of wet nappies or loose stools, or in the pattern of sleep, restlessness, crying or colic between infants in the two groups. The authors interpreted the lack of conclusive findings as signifying that no one pattern was better than the other and so the baby's appetite should determine whether they take one breast or two.

Discussion As with 'milk insufficiency', the reaction to inconsolable crying or colic will involve a combination of physical, psychological and social factors, which will be difficult to disentangle. There is little evidence to guide practice in this area. This is an important problem, however, which has the potential to cause huge disruption and distress to the family.

PRACTICE IMPLICATIONS:

- Professionals must help to enable women achieve effective positioning and attachment of the baby at the breast, as one of two key steps to ensure effective milk removal ('adequate breast emptying').

- Professionals should encourage women to feed for a prolonged period from each breast (or from one breast if the baby only wants one) to ensure the baby has an adequate opportunity to achieve effective milk removal.

- Women should have access to practical accurate support from appropriately trained professionals.

Further research Research is needed to examine further the hypothesis that changing feed management would reduce colic and distress in babies. The theoretical evidence is strong; a large clinical study, with good long-term follow up, would help to identify the numbers of babies who might respond to this treatment.

There is an urgent need to develop simple diagnostic tests for differentiating underfeeding from overfeeding for routine clinical use in the community.

Other causes of colic may include reactions to food the mother has eaten, or to additional food the baby may be receiving. This topic is outside the scope of this review, but a further review may identify the potential impact of this issue.

Research might help to examine treatment for babies, and their parents, who do not respond to changes in feed management. This may include non-pharmacological treatments such as massage, and support and education for parents.

6.4 Down's syndrome

Only one research study was identified on this topic. Aumonier and Cunningham (1983 [117]) interviewed 59 mothers of babies with chromosomally-confirmed Down's syndrome. Twenty nine women (54%) planned to breastfeed before birth. Six women (11%) were undecided; all started to bottle feed. Twenty six women actually started to breastfeed; of these, 16 breastfed for more than a month. None of the mothers reported that their baby's Down's syndrome was a cause for failure, although one mother reported that the hospital staff had discouraged her from breastfeeding when the Down's syndrome was diagnosed; 'insufficient milk' supply was given as the main reason for discontinuing breastfeeding. Only four of these mothers had babies who had sucking difficulties. Other problems encountered included an increased incidence of jaundice (49% of the total sample), and cardiac abnormalities (47% of the total sample). There was a significant relationship between initial sucking difficulties and severe cardiac abnormalities.

Discussion This paper demonstrates that it is possible for mothers of babies with Down's syndrome to breastfeed. Whether or not they succeed is likely to be affected by the encouragement or discouragement that they receive, and whether or not the baby has a serious cardiac abnormality.

PRACTICE IMPLICATIONS:

- Mothers will need practical accurate support from appropriately skilled professionals to establish and maintain successful and effective breastfeeding.

- Parents and other family members will need encouragement and support from the social network, in particular from other parents who have experience of the same circumstances.

- Parents should be put in direct contact with specialist lay groups capable of providing essential, accurate background knowledge and empathic support (e.g. Down's Association).

Further research Research in this area is difficult, as a result of the relatively small number of babies available to study. At the least, however, a series of case studies of babies with Down's syndrome whose mothers breastfeed would help to describe some of the problems and some of the possible solutions.

6.5 Cleft lip and palate

Cleft lip and palate are congenital malformations which result in incomplete fusing of the central processes around the upper jaw and lip. The cleft may involve only the lip, or it may extend into the hard and soft palate. It may be unilateral or bilateral. Treatment is surgical repair. Feeding at the breast is often difficult or impossible before repair, depending on the size of the lesion (Riordan & Auerbach 1993).

Two papers were identified which examined breastfeeding in relation to cleft lip. No studies examined babies with cleft palate.

In a descriptive study of 60 mothers and babies (Weatherley-White et al 1987 [118]), women were encouraged to breastfeed their babies immediately following surgical repair. Sixteen continued to breastfeed for six weeks or more, 22 were fed by cup or syringe, and 22 stopped breastfeeding in the six weeks after surgery. No complications attributable to breastfeeding were observed. Babies who were breastfed gained weight faster and went home earlier than those who were cup or syringe fed, but because this was not a randomised trial it is not possible to attribute cause and effect.

Darzi et al (1996 [119]) randomly assigned 40 infants with cleft lip alone to be either breastfed or spoon fed following surgical repair of the cleft. There were no differences in surgical outcome between the two groups although infants in the spoon fed group required more analgesia and i.v. fluids as they tended to be more irritable when breastfeeds were withheld. The authors support the view that breastfeeding should be promoted after cleft lip repair.

Discussion This challenging area affects a small number of babies, but it has a major impact on their ability to breastfeed successfully. Both studies (Weatherley-White et al 1987 [118], Darzi et al 1996 [119] suggest that with good care and support to breastfeed it is possible for babies to breastfeed after surgical repair of a cleft lip. A well established milk ejection reflex will help women to breastfeed a baby with a cleft lip or palate; so, such women will need a harmonious, relaxed and supportive environment in which to feed. Professionals should both work to help achieve this and offer encouragement to women while assisting them with breastfeeding.

PRACTICE IMPLICATIONS:

- Mothers of babies with a cleft lip are able to breastfeed and will need practical accurate support from appropriately skilled professionals.

- Babies with a cleft palate may be assisted to breastfeed with the aid of a prosthesis (palatal obdurator) prior to surgery.

- Breastfeeding is both possible and beneficial following surgical repair of a cleft lip and/or palate, and mothers will need practical accurate support from appropriately skilled professionals.

- Specialist medical and surgical teams dealing with these problems should employ an appropriately skilled health professional to whom all women have ready access.

- Professionals should be able to assist women with the establishment and management of milk expression in order to sustain an adequate milk supply.

- Mothers of babies with a cleft lip and/or palate will need encouragement and support from the social network with their feeding and will benefit from contact with, and support from specialist lay groups (e.g. Cleft Lip and Palate Association – CLAPA)

Further research Like Down's syndrome, this area is difficult to study as a result of the small numbers of babies affected. Again, a series of case studies would help to describe problems and possible solutions. It would be important to examine ways of supporting women who wish to express breastmilk until their baby has had surgery, and then to support them in the establishment of successful breastfeeding.

6.6 Tongue tie (ankyloglossia)

A baby with a short frenulum which inhibits extension of the tongue may have difficulty in grasping and maintaining an adequate mouthful of breast tissue. This may result in pain, sometimes severe, for the mother, and the baby receiving an inadequate milk supply. Treatment of the condition involves simple frenotomy, or cutting of the frenulum (Marmet et al 1990 [120]). The procedure is rapid and involves minimal blood loss. An alternative school of thought maintains that either the tongue will grow, or the frenulum will extend (or tear spontaneously) so that feeding will become more effective over time. There is little evidence either for the efficacy of this route or for what its time course might be.

No information is available about the prevalence of the condition. Anecdotal reports suggest that the condition is not uncommon, but may often go unrecognised.

Only two studies were identified which addressed this problem, both of which reported case studies (Marmet et al 1990 [120], Notestine 1990 [121]). A total of 15 cases are described in the two papers in which severe nipple and breast pain and slow growth in babies were associated with a tight frenulum in the baby. Frenotomy was performed in 9 of these babies, and resulted in pain-free, successful breastfeeding in all cases. No complications of the procedure were noted.

Discussion This condition, which can result in severe pain for the mother and growth problems for the baby, appears to have a relatively straightforward solution. There is a dearth of information, however, on it's definition, prevalence, treatment and possible side effects. It is likely that a proportion of the women who abandon breastfeeding because of nipple pain and trauma, or because of 'insufficient milk', may have babies with this condition. If the treatment is as effective and simple as is suggested, this discontinuation could be prevented.

Frenotomy appears to have been a relatively common procedure until the middle decades of this century, when breastfeeding became much less common. In the UK it has little credence with the medical profession as a therapeutic procedure to alleviate breastfeeding problems, although in Australia, for example, its routine use is still common (M Minchin, J Neil, pers. comms.). Both the expertise of the person performing the surgery (midwife, obstetrician, paediatric surgeon, oral or dental surgeon) must be considered and their preference for anaesthetic during the procedure (local or general, chloral hydrate, or no anaesthetic) are critical to the decision as to whether to proceed with a frenotomy to alleviate problems of breastfeeding.

PRACTICE IMPLICATIONS:

- Caregivers must be trained to diagnose the problem and to assess both its severity and its likely impact on breastfeeding.

- Professionals will need to alert mothers to the fact that they will probably need to place greater emphasis on breastfeeding technique in order to avoid nipple soreness and that they will require practical accurate support from appropriately skilled professionals

- Adjunctive use of mechanical breast expression (hand or pump) may be necessary to maintain breast milk supply and professionals should offer women support and assistance with this.

Further research Research is needed to identify the prevalence of tongue tie. This should include defining the range of presentations and severity. It is likely that individual variability in the relationship between the baby's mouth and the mother's breast will affect the decision-making process; for example, a breast which is small and has reservoirs close to the nipple may be easier for a baby with tongue tie to grasp, than a large, full breast. Such descriptive work would identify the babies and mothers who might benefit from intervention. The possible benefits and side effects of frenotomy should then be explored. If it is as simple and effective as described, work will be needed to explore ways of influencing practice.

KEY PRACTICE AREA F

**Practising evidence-based care
in maternity units**

There remains a need for a continued easing of the situation which has applied on maternity units in the past whereby restrictive practices have been imposed on the breastfeeding mother and her infant. Such restrictions have tended to suppress or over-ride the natural regulatory mechanisms intrinsic to breastfeeding, in particular, the process by which milk supply is regulated by infant demand, through the expression of infant appetite-control.

The WHO/UNICEF 'Ten Steps to Successful Breastfeeding', which underpin the Baby Friendly Hospital Initiative, seek to promote practices which protect and promote breast-feeding, and which are supportive of the breastfeeding woman. Simultaneously the scheme seeks to eliminate practices which have an adverse impact on the establishment of breastfeeding, and those which are not supported by physiological research.

These practices fall into six basic categories:
- Entrench physiologically-based practice as hospital policy to ensure the unequivocal delivery of evidence-based care to clients.
- Ensure that hospital staff are: (a) trained appropriately to have the knowledge to implement policy, and (b) skilled appropriately to assist women with feeding their baby effectively from a technical standpoint.
- Ensure that pregnant women are aware of the benefits of breastfeeding, and are sufficiently knowledgeable to be able to feed their babies effectively.
- Ensure that those practices which can have a beneficial impact on breastfeeding success (e.g. early initiation of breastfeeding, 'baby-led feeding', and 'rooming-in') are implemented in maternity units.
- Ensure, also, that those practices which are detrimental to the successful establishment of breastfeeding (e.g. the unnecessary giving of artificial formula, a reliance on bottle, teats and pacifiers) are eliminated from maternity units.
- Ensure that breastfeeding women are put in contact with, and assured access to, mother-to-mother support groups on discharge from the maternity unit.

The research base for the 'Ten Steps' has been described by Vallenas & Savage (WHO 1998).

6.7 Summary of baby problems

The dearth of studies in this important field resulted in running repeat searches to check that papers had not been omitted. We have been unable to identify any other papers, and have concluded that exploration of baby-related problems which make breastfeeding difficult, or which may affect well-being and contentment of the baby, has been consistently neglected. This is not only the case in areas where the number of babies affected is relatively small, such as cleft lip and palate, but also in areas where very large numbers of mothers and babies are affected each year, such as crying and jaundice.

7 General discussion and future research priorities

The volume of research covered by this review might give the erroneous impression that there is sufficient firm evidence available to inform practice in this field. In fact, the most striking finding is the paucity of good, well-designed research to inform an area of health care which has profound short and long term effects on such large numbers of people. These gaps are especially apparent in relation to the leading causes of breastfeeding discontinuation; 'insufficient milk', and sore nipples and breasts.

Factors underlying the scarcity of relevant, high quality research include the following:
- studies have not addressed some of the key practical issues in the field
- many studies are too small to be useful, or are methodologically flawed
- studies examining biomedical questions seldom consider the fundamental contribution of support, information and advice, the effects of women's views and feelings, and the social and cultural context of breastfeeding
- most studies reviewed took place in a culture when breastfeeding practices and routines were such that a large proportion of problems were a result of mismanagement. As a result, some very simple questions have not been addressed.

Future research priorities would more effectively address the problems of breastfeeding if these factors were taken into account. A coordinated approach to planning future research would provide an effective mechanism for addressing such challenges. Such an approach could ensure methodological rigour, the coordination of large studies, and the establishment of networks which would be needed to run appropriate studies examining less common issues. There are a number of funding bodies concerned with research in this field, including the NHS R&D programme, the MRC, the ESRC, a range of major charities, and international agencies. A mechanism such as the MRC topic review, involving all relevant bodies, would be a good means to start such a coordinated process.

Detailed questions for future research are given throughout the text. In general, future research in this field would benefit from dividing important issues into two:

1. **Issues which are common and widespread, affecting large numbers of women and babies, such as engorgement, 'insufficient milk', sore nipples and crying babies.** It would be feasible to organise large, simple

studies to answer a number of key questions. Information summarised in this review could be used to guide whether or not the key research questions relate to

a) the need for further studies of prevention or treatment, or
b) the need for studies to examine ways of implementing the results of existing research in practice. In a number of areas, both types of questions need to be addressed.

2. **Issues which are much less common, but result in distress and discontinuation of breastfeeding.** These include, for example, feeding for babies with specific problems such as Down's syndrome and cleft lip and palate. There is very little research to guide practice in any of these areas. Research in these areas will require a coordinated, national approach, as the numbers of mothers and babies affected in each local area is relatively small. In future, if it becomes possible to identify women with problems such as serious milk insufficiency, engorgement, or sore nipples, which do not resolve with good management and support, such a coordinated approach will also be necessary.

From the information reviewed in this paper, the three research areas which need to be most urgently addressed are:

- **a programme of work on milk insufficiency**; this is needed to address the multifaceted nature of the problem, including physical, psychological, professional and social factors. This is the leading cause of breastfeeding discontinuation worldwide and a range of work is needed to address it appropriately, including both large trials and detailed physiological studies.

- **why is it difficult to change practice in areas where research has demonstrated potential dramatic improvements for mothers and babies, and what would help to support such change?** Areas where evidence is available, but women still encounter great difficulties include the prevention of sore nipples and of engorgement. Such studies should include all relevant health professionals, such as paediatricians, midwives, GPs, health visitors and obstetricians.

- **pain-free, effective feeding is fundamental to successful breastfeeding and research is urgently needed to examine training programmes for caregivers to educate them in this essential skill.** A series of descriptive studies to identify the prevalence, types and natural history of the development of sore nipples and breasts is needed. Such descriptive information is essential before developing trials of treatments.

In addition to these clinical questions other important issues should be addressed. An analysis of the costs associated with infant feeding and its problems would demonstrate the scale of the demands on the health service which result from the present situation, and would guide the Department of Health, the NHS Executive, purchasers, and funding agencies in deciding what priority to give these issues. This process would be informed by a full-scale risk-assessment analysis of the health benefits and risks associated with alternative methods of infant feeding and different types of milk given. Addressing these questions would require both a systematic review, and empirical studies to examine factors such as use of NHS resources in the short and long term.

In summary

Factors conspire to prevent mothers and babies in the UK from breastfeeding their babies for as long as they wish to, as a result both of iatrogenic problems and a lack of useful research. The evidence reviewed here demonstrates areas where evidence is available to inform practice, and areas where further research is needed.

A coordinated approach to practice and research, involving the full range of professionals who work with mothers and babies, and the agencies involved in funding research in this field, is needed to address this urgent problem. Such an approach has succeeded in other countries.

8 Summary of recommendations for future research

Urgent research areas

1. The beliefs and attitudes of health professionals need urgent investigation, if the information derived from research and research reviews is to filter through to professional practice.

2. Pain-free, effective feeding is fundamental to successful breastfeeding and research is urgently needed to examine training programmes for caregivers to educate them in this essential skill. A series of descriptive studies to identify the prevalence, types and natural history of the development of sore nipples and breasts is needed. For example,
- how many women with sore nipples are not helped by correcting positioning techniques?
- how often are sore nipples associated with signs of infection, or problems in the baby such as tongue tie?
- do women develop breast pain in the absence of sore nipples, or are they always associated?
- how many women experience deep breast pain during and after feeds?

Such descriptive information is essential before developing trials of treatments.

3. There are many urgent questions about 'insufficient milk' which need to be addressed:
- Work is needed to distinguish the different types of 'milk insufficiency', and to develop simple diagnostic tests for discriminating between them
- Do women who are anaemic, or who have a heavy blood loss at birth, have subsequent problems in milk production? If so, can they be alleviated?
- A programme of supportive care (such as that described by Mathur et al, 1992) should be tested in a randomised controlled trial. This could be carried out both for women with 'insufficient milk', and for women in need of additional support, such as women with babies in neonatal units.
- Would anti-dopamine drugs enhance lactation for women who also receive supportive care, and would they be of use to women separated from their babies?
- Treatments for 'insufficient milk' which are often advised include prolonged feeding from one breast at each feed, breast massage, and

supplementing babies with bottles when slow weight gain is the presenting problem. These could be evaluated in trials.

A coordinated programme of work is needed to address appropriately the inter-related physical, psychological, professional, social and cultural issues.

Important research areas

1. There are a number of important and unanswered questions about engorgement:

- What is the prevalence of engorgement at the moment, and what would the prevalence be if women were encouraged and supported in carrying out preventive measures?
- Does antenatal expression of colostrum help in the prevention of engorgement?
- Does the local application of cabbage leaves help, and if so, when and what are the best methods of using them?
- Would oral proteolytic enzymes help?
- Would a regime such as that used in the ultrasound trial, including warmth, rest, breast massage and practical information and support, help women with engorgement?
- Would simple breast support, in the form of a well-fitting bra or breast binder, together with analgesia, help women with painful engorgement?
- Engorged breasts can become very swollen and hard, making it difficult for the baby to attach well. Are there techniques which would help women whose breasts are very swollen and painful to enable the baby to attach well to the breast?
- Would warm baths/showers and gentle expression help?

Many of these questions could be effectively addressed in randomised controlled trials.

2. There is an important need to identify the prevalence of mastitis in this country, and the range of suggested treatments.

3. Methods for the identification of women suspected to have been the victims of sexual abuse and evaluation of the efficacy of counselling in such situations is a much-needed area for research.

4. The dearth of studies examining baby-related feeding problems resulted in running repeat searches to check that papers had not been omitted. We have been unable to identify any other papers, and have concluded that exploration of baby-related problems which make breastfeeding difficult, or which may affect well-being and contentment of the baby, has been consistently neglected. This is

not only the case in areas where the number of babies affected is relatively small, such as cleft lip and palate, but also in areas where very large numbers of mothers and babies are affected each year, such as crying and jaundice.

Costs associated with infant feeding and its problems

An analysis of the costs associated with infant feeding and its problems would demonstrate the scale of the demands on the health service which result from the present situation, and would guide the Department of Health, the NHS Executive, purchasers, and funding agencies in deciding what priority to give these issues. This process would be informed by a full-scale risk-assessment analysis of the health benefits and risks associated with alternative methods of infant feeding and different types of milk given. Addressing these questions would require both a systematic review, and empirical studies to examine factors such as use of NHS resources in the short and long term.

OVERVIEW OF PRACTICE IMPLICATIONS

- Mechanisms need to be in place to ensure that adverse attitudes against breastfeeding held by healthcare staff do not influence their interactions with women. It is especially necessary to observe this at the first point of contact between a pregnant women and her midwife to ensure that pregnant women are not discouraged from considering breastfeeding their infant.

- All healthcare workers having contact with women antenatally should have a clear knowledge of the health benefits of breastfeeding and familiarity with how to engage women in an informed discussion of the issues affecting their choice of feeding method.

- Antenatal education for pregnant women and their partners (and other family members who may be interested) should be addressed to ensure that the practical skills are taught effectively and that all family members understand the baby's normal pattern of behaviour (sleeping, crying, feeding).

- Midwives and other healthcare workers should have a sound physiological knowledge of the process underlying breast milk production and transfer, and of the relevance of this knowledge to clinical practice.

- Midwives and other healthcare workers should have the opportunity to develop the necessary skills, expertise and experience in assisting women with the essential breastfeeding skills of positioning and attachment of the baby at the breast, and of how to correct inappropriate practices.

- Midwives and other healthcare workers should receive training in counselling skills from experienced and competent personnel to ensure that they are consistently capable of supporting women and of offering assistance in an empathic and sensitive manner, thereby enabling women to develop the necessary breastfeeding skills for themselves. They should also have adequate opportunity to deliver those skills to the women and babies in their care.

- Education to increase awareness of all healthcare workers in the general issues surrounding the promotion and protection of breastfeeding, and with how to support the breastfeeding mother.

- Education of the general public to increase awareness of the benefits of breastfeeding, the realities of physiological breastfeeding, and the general response of the public at large to common problems of feeding infants and of parenting generally.

9 References

Adams J A, Hey D J & Hall R T. Incidence of hyperbilirubinemia in breast-vs. formula-fed infants. *Clinical Pediatrics*. 1985 Feb; **24(2)**:69–73. [Table 113]

Akre J (Ed.). Infant feeding: the physiological basis. Geneva: World Health Organization; 1989. 108 pp [citation from Chapter 3, p43]

Alexander J M, Grant A M, & Campbell M. J. Randomised controlled trial of breast shells and Hoffman's exercises for inverted and non-protractile nipples. *Brit Med J*. 1992 Apr 18; **304(6833)**:1030–2. [Table 12]

Allen L H, & Pelto G H. Research on determinants of breastfeeding duration: suggestions for biocultural studies. *Medical Anthropology*. 1986; **9**:97.

Amir L H, & Pakula S. Nipple pain, mastalgia and candidiasis in the lactating breast. *Australian & New Zealand Journal of Obstetrics & Gynaecology*. 1991 Nov; **31(4)**:378–80.

Amroth S G. Water requirements of breast-fed infants in a hot climate. *American Journal of Clinical Nutrition*. 1978; **31**:1154–1157.

Anderson G C. Current knowledge about skin-to-skin (kangaroo) care for preterm infants. [Review]. *Journal of Perinatology*. 1991 Sep; **11(3)**:216–26.

Anderson S, Shakya K N, Shrestha L N, & Costello A M. Hypoglycaemia: a common problem among uncomplicated newborn infants in Nepal. *Journal of Tropical Paediatrics*. 1993 Oct; **39(5)**:273–7.

Aono T, Aki T, Koike K, & Kurachi K. Effect of sulpiride on poor puerperal lactation. *American Journal of Obstetrics & Gynecology*. 1982 Aug 15; **143(8)**:927–32. [Table 102]

Aono T, Shioji T, Aki T, Hirota K, Nomura A, & Kurachi K. Augmentation of puerperal lactation by oral administration of sulpiride. *Journal of Clinical Endocrinology & Metabolism*. 1979 Mar; **48(3)**:478–82. [Table 101]

Ardran G M, Kemp F H, & Lind J. A cineradiographic study of breastfeeding. *British Journal of Radiology*. 1958; **31**:156–162.

Arnestad M, Anderson M, & Rognum T O. Is the use of dummy or carry-cot of importance for sudden infant death? *European Journal of Pediatrics*. 1998. **157(11)**:968–70.

Atkinson L D. Prenatal nipple conditioning for breastfeeding. *Nursing Research*. 1979; **28(5)**:267–271. [Table 7]

Auerbach K G. The effect of nipple shields on maternal milk volume. *Journal of Obstetric, Gynecologic, & Neonatal Nursing*. 1990 Sep; **19(5)**:419–27. [Table 67]

Auerbach K G, & Gartner L M. 'Breastfeeding and human milk : their association with jaundice in the neonate'. *Clinics in Perinatology.* 1987; **14**:89–107.

Auerbach K G, Renfrew M J, & Minchin M A. Infant feeding comparisons: A hazard to infant health? *Journal of Human Lactation.* 1991; **7**:63–71.

Aumonier M E, & Cunningham C C. Breast feeding in infants with Down's syndrome. *Child: Care, Health & Development.* 1983 Sep; **9(5)**:247–55. [Table 117]

Barros F C, Victora C G, Semer T C, Filho S T, Tomasi E, & Weiderpass E. Use of pacifiers is associated with decreased breast-feeding duration. *Pediatrics.* 1995; **95(4)**:497–9.

Barros F C, Victora C G, Morris S S, Halpern R, Horta B L, & Tomasi E. Breast feeding, pacifier use and infant development at 12 months of age: a birth cohort study in Brazil. *Paediatric & Perinatal Epidemiology.* 1997; **11(4)**:441–50.

Bauchner H, Leventhal J M, & Shapiro E D. Studies of breast-feeding and infections. How good is the evidence? [Review]. *JAMA.* 1986 Aug 15; **256(7)**:887–92.

Baumslag N, & Michels D L. Milk, money and madness: the culture and politics of breastfeeding. Westport, Connecticut: Bergin and Garvey; 1995.

Beekman D. "The Mechanical Baby". First ed. New York: Meridian; 1977.

Bergevin Y, Dougherty C, & Kramer M S. Do infant formula samples shorten the duration of breastfeeding? *The Lancet.* 1983; 1148–1151. [Table 57]

Bernard-Bonnin A C, Stachtchenko S, Girard G, & Rousseau E. Hospital practices and breastfeeding duration: a meta-analysis of controlled trials. *Birth.* 1989; **16(2)**:64–6.

Blaikeley J, Clarke S, Mackeith R, & Ogden K M. Breastfeeding: factors affecting success. *Journal of Obstetrics and Gynaecology of the British Empire.* 1953; **60**:657–669. [Table 2]

Bliss M C, Wilkie J, Acredolo C, Berman S, & Tebb K P. The effect of discharge pack formula and breast pumps on breastfeeding duration and choice of infant feeding method. *Birth.* 1997; **24(2)**:90–7. [Table 63]

Blomquist H K, Jonsbo F, Serenius F, & Persson L A. Supplementary feeding in the maternity ward shortens the duration of breast feeding. *Acta Paediatrica.* 1994; **83(11)**:1122–6. [Table 54]

van den Bosch C A, & Bullough C H W. Effect of early suckling on term neonates' core body temperature. *Annals of Tropical Paediatrics.* 1990; **10(4)**:347–353. [Table 20]

Bosma J F, Hepburn L G, Josell S D, & Baker K. Ultrasound demonstration of tongue motions during suckle feeding. *Developmental Medicine and Child Neurology.* 1990; **32**:223–9.

Brown G L, Nanney L B, Griffen J, Cramer A B, Yancey J M, Curtsinger L J, Holtzin L, Schultz G S, Jurkiewicz M J, & Lynch J B. Enhancement of wound healing by topical treatment with epidermal growth factor. *The New*

England Journal of Medicine. 1989; **321(2)**:76–9.

Brown K H, Black R E, Robertson A D, Akhtar N A, Ahmed G, & Becker S. Clinical and field studies of human lactation: methodological considerations. *American Journal of Clinical Nutrition.* 1982; 745–756.

Brown K H, Creed de Kanashiro H, Aguila R, Lopez de Romana G, & Black R. Milk consumption and hydration status of exclusively breastfed infants in a warm climate. *Pediatrics.* 1986; **108**:677–680.

Brown M S & Hurlock J T. Preparation of the breast for breastfeeding. *Nursing Research.* 1975; **24(6)**:448–451. [Table 4]

Bu'Lock F, Woolridge M W & Baum J D. Development of coordination of sucking, swallowing and breathing: ultrasound study of term and preterm infants. *Developmental Medicine and Child Neurology.* 1990; **32**: 669–78.

Buchko B L, Pugh L C, Bishop B A, Cochran J F, Smith L R, & Lerew D J. Comfort measures in breastfeeding, primiparous women. *Journal of Obstetric, Gynecologic, & Neonatal Nursing.* 1993; **23(1)**:46–52. [Table 36]

de Carvalho M, Hall M, & Harvey D. Effects of water supplementation on physiological jaundice in breast-fed babies. *Archives of Disease in Childhood.* 1981; **56(7)**:568–9. [Table 47]

de Carvalho M, Klaus M H, & Merkatz R B. Frequency of breast-feeding and serum bilirubin concentration. *American Journal of Disease of Childhood.* 1982; **136**:737–8. [Table 114]

de Carvalho M, Robertson S, & Klaus M H. Does the duration and frequency of early breastfeeding affect nipple pain?. *Birth: Issues in Perinatal Care & Education.* 1984 Apr–1984; **11(2)**:81–4. [Table 40]

de Carvalho M, Robertson S, Friedman A, & Klaus M. Effect of frequent breastfeeding on early milk production and infant weight gain. *Pediatrics.* 1983; **72(3)**:307–311. [Table 41]

de Chateau P, Holmberg H, Jakobsson K, & Winberg J. A study of factors promoting and inhibiting lactation. *Developmental Medicine & Child Neurology.* 1977; **19(5)**:575–84. [Table 27]

Casey C E, Neifert M R, Seacat J M, & Neville M C. Nutrient intake by breastfed infants during the first five days after birth. *American Journal of Diseases of Childhood.* 1986; **140**:933–936.

Clark M. A study of four methods of nipple care offered to post partum mothers. *The New Zealand Journal of Medicine.* 1985; 16–18. [Table 9]

Cornblath M, Schwartz R, Aynsley-Green A, & Lloyd J K. Hypoglycaemia in infancy: the need for a rational definition. *Pediatrics.* 1990; **85**:834–7.

Cronenwett L, Stukel T, Kearney M, Barrett J, Covington C, Del Monte K, Reinhardt R, & Rippe L. Single daily bottle use in the early weeks postpartum and breast-feeding outcomes. *Pediatrics.* 1992; **90(5)**:760–6. [Table 50]

Culley P, Milan P, Roginski C, Waterhouse J, & Wood B. Are breast-fed babies still getting a raw deal in hospital? *British Medical Journal.* 1979 **2(6195)**:891–3.

Cunningham A S. Studies of breastfeeding and infections. How good is the evidence? A critique of the answer from Yale. *Journal of Human Lactation.* 1988; **4**:54–56.

Cunningham A S, Jelliffe D B, & Jelliffe E F P. Breastfeeding, Growth and Illness: An Annotated Bibliography. 1992; New York: UNICEF.

Daly S E J, Kent J C, Huynh D Q, Owens R A, Alexander B F, Ng K C, & Hartmann P E. The determination of short-term breast volume changes and the rate of synthesis of human milk using computerised breast measurement. *Experimental Physiology.* 1992; **77**:79–87.

Daly S E J, Kent J C, Owens R A, & Hartmann P E. Frequency and degree of milk removal and the short-term control of human milk synthesis. *Experimental Physiology.* 1996; **81 (5)**:861–75.

Daly S E J, Owens R A, & Hartmann P E. The Short-term Synthesis and Infant-Regulated Removal of Milk in Lactating Women. *Experimental Physiology.* 1993; **78**:209–220.

Darzi M A, Chowdri N A, & Bhat A N. Breast feeding or spoon feeding after cleft lip repair: a prospective, randomised study. *British Journal of Plastic Surgery.* 1996; **49**:24–6. [Table 119]

Darwazeh A M, & al-Bashir A. Oral candidal flora in healthy infants. *Journal of Oral Pathology & Medicine.* 1995; **24(8)**:361–4.

Dearlove J C, & Dearlove B M. Prolactin, fluid balance and lactation. *British Journal of Obstetrics & Gynaecology.* 1981 Jun; **88(6)**:652–4. [Table 92]

Department of Health. Breastfeeding: Good Practice Guidance to the NHS. 1995 May. Prepared in consultation with National Breastfeeding Working Group.

Devereux W P. Acute puerperal mastitis. Evaluation of its management. American *Journal of Obstetrics & Gynecology.* 1969 Sep 1; **108(1)**:78–81. [Table 85]

Dewey K G, & Lonnerdal B. Infant self-regulation of breast-milk intake. *Acta Paediatrica Scandinavica.* 1986; **75**:893–8.

Dewey K G, Heinig M J, Nommsen L A, & Lonnerdal B. Adequacy of energy intake among breastfed infants in the DARLING study. *Journal of Pediatrics.* 1991; **119**:538–47.

Donnelly A, Renfrew M J, Woolridge M W, Martin L A, Snowden H M. The influence of discharge packs on the duration and exclusivity of breastfeeding (Protocol). The Cochrane Library, Issue 1, 2000. Update Software, Oxford, UK.

Drane D, Fernandez A, & Minchin M. Literature review on breast milk expression, storage, and feeding. Washington, D.C.: Wellstart International; 1994.

Drewett R F, Woolridge M W, Jackson D A, Imong S M, Mangklabruks A, Wongsawasdii L, Chiowanich P, Amatayakul K, & Baum J D. Relationships between nursing patients, supplementary food intake and breast-milk intake in a rural Thai population. *Early Human Development*, 1989, **20**:13–23.

Drewett R, Amatayakul K, Wongsawasdii L, Mangklabruks A, Ruckpaopunt S, Ruangyuttikarn C, Baum D, Imong S, Jackson D, & Woolridge M. Nursing frequency and the energy intake from breast milk and supplementary food in a rural Thai population: a longitudinal study. *European Journal of Clinical Nutrition*. 1993; **47**:880–891.

Duffy E P, Percival P, & Kershaw E. Positive effects of an antenatal group teaching session on postnatal nipple pain, nipple trauma and breast feeding rates. *Midwifery*. 1997; **13**:189–96. [Table 31]

Duncan B, Ey J, Holberg C J, Wright A L, Martinez F D, & Taussig L M. Exclusive breastfeeding for at least four months protects against otitis media. *Pediatrics*. 1993; **91(5)**:867–72.

Dungy C I, Christensen-Szalanski J, Losch M, & Russell D. Effect of discharge samples on duration of breast-feeding [see comments]. *Pediatrics*. 1992 Aug; **90(2 Pt 1)**:233–7. [Table 61]

Dungy C I, Losch M E, Russell D, Romitti P, & Dusdieker L B. Hospital infant formula discharge packages. *Archives of Paediatric and Adolescent Medicine*. 1997; **151**:724–9. [Table 64]

Egli G E, Egli N S, & Newton M. The influence of the number of breast feedings on milk production. *Pediatrics* 1961; **27**:314–7.

Ehrenkranz R A, & Ackerman B A. Metoclopramide effect on faltering milk production by mothers of premature infants. *Pediatrics*. 1986; **78(4)**:614–620.

Eiger M S, & Olds S W. The Complete Book of Breastfeeding. New York: Workman Publishing; 1987.

Elander G, & Lindberg T. Hospital routines in infants with hyperbilirubinemia influence the duration of breast feeding. *Acta Paediatrica Scandinavica*. 1986; **75**:708–712. [Table 115]

Eppink H. An experiment to determine a basis for nursing decisions in regard to time of initiation of breastfeeding. *Nursing Research*. 1969, **18(4)**:292–9. [Table 18]

l'Esperance, C M. Pain or pleasure: the dilemma of early breastfeeding. *Birth Family Journal*. 1980; **7**:21–26. [Table 11]

Evans C J, Lyons N B, & Killien M G. The effect of infant formula samples on breastfeeding practice. *Journal of Obstetric, Gynaecologic, and Neonatal Nursing*. 1986; **15**:401–405. [Table 59]

Evans K, Evans R, & Simmer K. Effect of the method of breast feeding on breast engorgement, mastitis and infantile colic. *Acta Paediatrica*. 1995 Aug; **84(8)**:849–52. [Table 73]

Faculty of Public Health Medicine. 'Promoting Breastfeeding'. Guidelines for Health Promotion Number 41. Royal College of Physicians of the United Kingdom. 1995.

Feinstein J M, Berkelhamer J E, Gruszka M E, Wong C A, and Carey A E.

Factors related to early termination of breastfeeding in an urban population. *Paediatrics*. 1986; **78(2)**:210–215. [Table 60]

Fisher C. On demand breastfeeding: Aspects of Midwifery. *Midwife Health Visitor & Community Nurse*. 1986 Jun; **22**:194–198.

Fleming P A. The effect of prenatal nipple conditioning on postpartum nipple pain of breastfeeding women. *Health Care for Women International*. 1984, **5**:453–7. [Table 8]

Fleming P J, Blair P S, Bacon C, Bensley D, Smith I, Taylor E, Berry J, Golding J, Tripp J, et al. Environment of infants during sleep and risk of the sudden infant death syndrome: results of 1993–5 case-control study for confidential inquiry into stillbirths and deaths in infancy. *British Medical Journal*. 1996; **213**:191–5.

Fomon S J, Filer L J, Thomas T A, Anderson, T A, & Nelson S E. Influence of formula concentration on caloric intake and growth of normal infants. *Acta Paediatrica Scandinavica*. 1975; **75**:893–898.

Foster K, Lader D, & Cheesbrough S. Infant Feeding 1995. London: The Stationery Office; 1997.

Foxman B, Schwartz K, & Looman S J. Breastfeeding practice and lactation mastitis. *Social Science & Medicine*. 1994 Mar; **38(5)**:755–761. [Table 83]

Frank D A, Wirtz S J, Sorenson J R, & Heeren T. Commercial discharge packs and breastfeeding counselling: effects on infants feeding practices in a randomised trial. *Pediatrics*. 1987; **80(6)**:845–854. [Table 58]

Freed G L, Clark S J, Sorenson J, Lohr J A, Cefalo R, & Curtis P. National assessment of physicians' breastfeeding knowledge, attitudes, training and experience. *JAMA*. 1995; **273(6)**:472–476.

Friedman E A, & Sachtleben M R. Oxytocin in lactation. *American Journal of Obstetrics and Gynaecology*. 1961; **82**:846–855.

Gale C R, & Martyn C N. Breastfeeding, dummy use, and adult intelligence. *The Lancet*. 1996; **347(9008)**:1072–5.

Gale R, Dollberg S, Branski D, Stevenson D K, & Seidman D S. Breastfeeding term infants. *Clinical Pediatrics*. 1989; **28(10)**:458–460. [Table 42]

Gangal H T, & Gangal M H. Suction method for correcting flat nipples or inverted nipples. *Plastic & Reconstructive Surgery*. 1978; **61**:294–6.

Garcia J, Redshaw M, Fitzsimmons B & Keene J. First class delivery: A national survey of women's views of maternity care. National Perinatal Epidemiology Unit. Audit Commission, 1998; 109pp.

Garforth S, & Garcia J. Breastfeeding policies in practice – No wonder they get confused. *Midwifery*. 1989; **5**:75–83.

de Gezelle H, Ooghe W, Thiery M, & Dhont M. Metoclopramide and breast milk. *European Journal of Obstetrics, Gynecology, & Reproductive Biology*. 1983 Apr; **15(1)**:31–6. [Table 100]

Girija A, Geervani P, & Nageswara Rao G. Influence of dietary supplementation during lactation on lactation performance. *Journal of Tropical Pediatrics*. 1984 Jun; **30**:140–144.

Gokhale M. A herbal drug that stimulates lactation. *Indian Practitioner.* 1965 Sep; **18(9)**:665–670. [Table 111]

Goldberg N M, & Adams E. Supplementary water for breast-fed babies in a hot and dry climate-not really a necessity. *Archives of Disease in Childhood.* 1983; **58**:514–518.

Gosha J L, & Tichy A M. Effect of a breast shell on postpartum nipple pain: an exploratory study. *Journal of Nurse-Midwifery.* 1988 Mar; **33(2)**:74–7. [Table 70]

Gray R H, Campbell O M, Apelo R, Eslami S S, Zacur H, Ramos R M, Gehret J C, & Labbok M H. Risk of ovulation during lactation. *The Lancet.* 1990; **335**:25–9.

Gray-Donald K, Kramer M S, Munday S, and Leduc D G. Effect of formula supplementation in the hospital on the duration of breastfeeding. *Pediatrics.* 1985; **75**:514–518. [Table 53]

Green J M, Coupland V A, & Kitzinger J V. "Great Expectations: A prospective study of women's expectations and experiences of childbirth." Books for Midwives Press, Cheshire, England, 1998.

Gregg J E. Attitudes of teenagers in Liverpool to breast feeding. *British Medical Journal.* 1989; **299(6692)**:147–148.

Gunther M. "Infant Feeding". Chicago: Henry Regenery Company; 1970.

Gunther M. Sore nipples: causes and prevention. Lancet. 1945; **ii**: 590–593. [Table 29]

Guthrie G M, Guthrie H A, Fernandez T L, Estrera N O. Infant formula samples and breastfeeding among Philippine urban poor. *Soc. Sci. Med.* 1985; **20(7)**:713–7.

Guzman V, Toscano G, Canales E S, and Zarate A. Improvement of defective lactation by using oral metoclopramide. *Acta Obstetrica et Gynecologica Scandinavica.* 1979; **58**:53–55. [Table 95]

Hamosh M, & Goldman A S. Human Lactation 2: Maternal and Environmental Factors. New York: Plenum Press; 1986.

Hardyment C. Dream Babies. London: Cape; 1983.

Hawdon J M, et al. Patterns of neonatal adaptation for preterm and term infants in the first neonatal week. *Archives of Disease in Childhood.* 1992; **68**:357–65.

Hawdon J M, Platt M P, and Aynsley-Green A. Neonatal hypoglycaemia – blood glucose monitoring and baby feeding. *Midwifery.* 1993 Mar; **9(1)**:3–6.

Hawken J. Unpublished observations. 1982.

Heck I J, & Erenberg. Serum glucose levels in term neonates during the first 48 hours of life. *Journal of Pediatrics.* 1987; **110**:119–122.

Helsing E, and Kjaernes U. A Silent Revolution – Changes in Maternity Ward Routines with Regard to Infant Feeding in Norway 1973–1982. *Acta Paediatr Scand.* 1985; **74**:332–337.

Henly S J, Anderson C M, Avery M D, Hills-Bonczyk S G, Potter S, and

Duckett L J. Anemia and insufficient milk in first-time mothers. *Birth: Issues in Perinatal Care & Education.* 1995 Jun; **22(2)**:87–92. [Table 88]

Herd B, & Feeney J G. Two aerosol sprays in nipple trauma. *Practitioner.* 1986; **230**:31–38. [Table 33]

Hewat R J and Ellis D J. A comparison of the effectiveness of two methods of nipple care. *Birth: Issues in Perinatal Care & Education.* 1987 Mar; **14(1)**:41–5. [Table 5]

Hill P D. Insufficient milk supply syndrome. *NAACOGS Clinical Issues in Perinatal & Womens Health Nursing.* 1992; **3(4)**:605–12.

Hill P D, & Aldag J. Potential indicators of insufficient milk supply syndrome. *Research in Nursing & Health.* 1991 Feb; **14(1)**:11–9.

Hillervik-Lindquist C. Studies on perceived breast milk insufficiency. A prospective study in a group of Swedish women. *Acta Paediatrica Scandinavica.* Suppl. 1991; **376**:1–27. [Table 94]

Hinman C D, & Mailbach H. Effect of air exposure and occlusion on experimental human skin wounds. *Nature.* 1963; **200**:377–88.

Hofmeyr G J, van Iddekinge B, and Blott J A. Domperidone: secretion in breastmilk and effect on puerperal prolactin levels. *British Journal of Obstetrics and Gynaecology.* 1985; **92**:141–144. [Table 106]

Host A H, Husby S & Osterballe O. A prospective study of cow's milk allergy in exclusively breast-fed infants. *Acta Paediatr. Scand.* 1988; **77**:663–70.

Host A, Husby S, Gjesing B, Larsen J N, and Lowenstein H. Prospective estimation of IgG, IgG subclass and IgE antibodies to dietary proteins in infants with cow milk allergy. Levels of antibodies to whole milk protein, BLG and ovalbumin in relation to repeated milk challenge and clinical course of cow milk allergy. *Allergy.* 1992; **47(3)**:218–229.

Houston M J. Home support for the breast feeding mother. Maternal and Infant Health Care. First ed. Edinburgh: Churchill Livingstone; 1984.

Houston M J, Howie P W, Cook A, and McNeilly A S. Do breast feeding mothers get the home support they need?. *Health Bulletin.* 1981 May; **39(3)**:166–72.

Houston M J, Howie P W, and McNeilly A S. Factors affecting the duration of breast feeding: 1. Measurement of breast milk intake in the first week of life. *Early Human Development.* 1983a; **8(1)**:49–54.

Houston M J, Howie P W, Smart L, McArdle T, and McNeilly A S. Factors affecting the duration of breast feeding: 2. Early feeding practices and social class. *Early Human Development.* 1983b; **8(1)**:55–63. [Table 90]

Houston M, Howie P W, and McNeilly A S. The effect of extra fluid intake by breastfed babies in hospital on the duration of breastfeeding. Comparison of 3 regimes on different wards. *Journal of Reproductive and Infant Psychology.* 1984; **2**:42–48. [Table 52]

Howard C R, Howard F M, Lanphear B, de Blieck E A, Eberly S, & Lawrence R A. The effects of early pacifier use on breastfeeding duration. *Pediatrics.* 1999; **103(3)**:E33.

Howie P W, Forsyth J S, Ogston S A, Clark A, and Florey C du V. Protective effect of breastfeeding against infection. *British Medical Journal.* 1990; **300**:11–16.

Howie P W, Houston M J, Cook A, Smart L, McArdle T, and McNeilly A S. How long should a breast feed last?. *Early Human Development.* 1981 Feb; **5(1)**:71–7. [Table 43]

Huggins K E, & Billon S F. Twenty cases of persistent sore nipples: collaboration between lactation consultant and dermatologist. *Journal of Human Lactation.* 1993 Sep; **9(3)**:155–60. [Table 72]

Huntingford P J. Intranasal use of synthetic oxytocin in management of breastfeeding. *British Medical Journal.* 1961; **2**:709–711.

Hytten F E. Clinical and chemical studies in human lactation. *British Medical Journal.* 1954; **1**:175–182.

Illingworth R S, Stone D G H, Jowett G H, and Scott J F. Self-demand feeding in a maternity unit. *The Lancet.* 1952; **1**:683–7. [Table 39]

Inch S. Unpublished observations. 1980.

Inch S, & Fisher C. Mastitis: infection or inflammation?. [Review]. *Practitioner.* 1995 Aug; **239(1553)**:472–6. [Table 84]

Inch S, & Garforth S. Establishing and maintaining breastfeeding. Chalmers I, Enkin M W, and Keirse M, Editors. Effective care in pregnancy and childbirth. Oxford: Oxford University Press; 1989; pp. 1359–74.

Inch S, & Renfrew M J. Common breastfeeding problems. Chalmers I, Enkin M W, and Keirse M, Editors. Effective care in pregnancy and childbirth. Oxford: Oxford University Press; 1989; p. 1375.

Ingelman-Sundberg A. The value of antenatal massage of nipples and expression of colostrum. *Journal of Obstetrics and Gynaecology of the British Empire.* 1958; **65**:448–449. [Table 3]

Jenner S. The influence of additional information, advice and support on the success of breastfeeding in the working class primiparas. *Child: Care, Health & Development.* 1988; **14**:319–28.

Johnson C A, Lieberman B, & Hassanein R E. The relationship of breastfeeding to third day bilirubin levels. *Journal of Family Practice.* 1985; **20(2)**:147–152. [Table 48]

Johnson N W. Breast-feeding at one hour of age. *American Journal of Maternal and Child Nursing (MCN).* 1976, **Jan/Feb**: 12–16. [Table 23]

Jonsson S, & Pulkkinen M O. Mastitis today: incidence, prevention and treatment. *Annales Chirurgiae et Gynaecologiae* Supplementum. 1994; **208**:84–87. [Table 80]

Kaufmann R, & Foxman B. Mastitis among lactating women: occurrence and risk factors. *Social Science & Medicine.* 1991; **33(6)**:701–5. [Table 81]

Kauppila A, Kivinen S, & Ylikorkala O. A dose response relation between improved lactation and metoclopramide. *The Lancet.* 1981a; **i**:1175–7. [Table 97]

Kauppila A, Kivinen S, & Ylikorkala O. Metoclopramide increases prolactin release and milk secretion in puerperium without stimulating the secretion of thyrotropin and thyroid hormones. *Journal of Clinical Endocrinology and Metabolism*. 1981b; **52**:436–9. [Table 98]

Kauppila A, Anunti P, Kivinen S, Koivisto M, & Ruokonen A. Metoclopramide and breast feeding: efficacy and anterior pituitary responses of the mother and the child. *European Journal of Obstetrics, Gynecology, & Reproductive Biology*. 1988; **19(1)**:19–22. [Table 99]

Kee W H, Tan S L, Lee V, and Salmon Y M. The treatment of breast engorgement with serrapeptase (Danzen): a randomised double-blind controlled trial. *Singapore Medical Journal*. 1989 **Feb; 30(1)**:48–54. [Table 79]

Kennedy K, Rivera R, & McNeilly A. Consensus statement on the use of breast-feeding as a family planning method. *Contraception*. 1989; **39(5)**:477–96.

Kesaree N, Banapurmath C R, Banapurmath S, & Shamanur K. Treatment of inverted nipples using a disposable syringe. *Journal of Human Lactation*. 1993; **9(1)**:27–9. [Table 15]

Koh T H H G, Aynsley-Green A, Tarbit M, & Eyre J. Neural dysfunction during hypoglycaemia. *Archives of Disease of Childhood*. 1988; **63**: 1353–58.

Kurinij N, & Shiono P H. Early formula supplementation of breast-feeding. *Pediatrics*. 1991; **88(4)**:745–9.

Lavergne N A. Does application of tea bags to sore nipples while breastfeeding provide effective relief. *Journal of Obstetric, Gynecologic, & Neonatal Nursing*. 1997; **26(1)**:53–7. [Table 38]

Lawrence R A. Breastfeeding: a guide for the medical profession. Fourth ed. St Louis: Mosby; 1994.

Lewis P J, Devenish C, & Kahn C. Controlled trial of metoclopramide in the initiation of breast-feeding. *British Journal of Clinical Pharmacology*. 1980; **9**:217–9. [Table 96]

Long L. Breastfeeding workshops: a focus on knowledge, skills and attitudes. *British Journal of Midwifery*. 1995; **3(10)**:540–4.

Lucas A, Brooke O G, Morley R, Cole T J, & Bamford M F. Early diet of preterm infants and development of allergic or atopic disease: randomised prospective study. *British Medical Journal*. 1990; **300**:837–40.

Lucas A, Lockton S & Davies P S W. Randomised trial of a ready-to-feed compared with powdered formula. *Archives of Disease of Childhood*. 1992; **67**:935–39.

Luhman L A. The effect of intranasal oxytocin on lactation. *Obstetrics and Gynaecology*. 1963; **21**:713–717.

The MAIN Trial Collaborative Group . Preparing for breast feeding: treatment of inverted and non-protractile nipples in pregnancy. *Midwifery*. 1994 Dec; **10(4)**:200–14. [Table 13]

Marmet C, Shell E, & Marmet R. Neonatal frenotomy may be necessary to correct breastfeeding problems. *Journal of Human Lactation*. 1990 Sep; **6(3)**:117–21. [Table 120]

Marshall B R, Hepper J K, & Zirbel C C. Sporadic puerperal mastitis. An infection that need not interrupt lactation. *JAMA*. 1975 Sep 29; **233(13)**:1377–9.

Martin J, & Monk J. Infant feeding 1980. Office of Population Census and Surveys, Social Survey Division. London: Her Majesty's Stationery Office; 1982.

Martin J, & White A. Infant feeding 1985. Office of Population Census and Surveys, Social Survey Division. London: Her Majesty's Stationery Office; 1988.

Martin L A, Renfrew M J, Woolridge M W. Additional food and fluids for breastfed infants (protocol). The Cochrane Library 1999; Issue 2. Update Software, Oxford, UK.

Martin-Calama J, Buñuel J, Valero T, Labay M, Lasarte J J, Valle F, & de Miguel C. The effect of feeding glucose water to breastfeeding newborns on weight, body temperature, blood glucose, and breastfeeding duration. *Journal of Human Lactation*. 1997; **13(3)**:209–13. [Table 51]

Martindale. The extra pharmacopoeia. 28th ed. London: London Pharmaceutical Press; 1982.

Martinez J C, Maisels M J, Otheguy L, Garcia H, Savorani M, Mogni B, and Martinez J C jnr. Hyperbilirubinemia in the breast-fed newborn: a controlled trial of four interventions. *Pediatrics*. 1993; **91(2)**:470–473. [Table 46]

Mathur G P, Chitranshi S, Mathur S, Singh S B, & Bhalla M. Lactation failure. *Indian Pediatrics*. 1992 Dec; **29(12)**:1541–4. [Table 93]

Matthew W H, Taylor B, Norman A P, Turner M W, & Soothill J F. Prevention of eczema. *The Lancet*. 1977; **1**:321–324.

McGeorge D D. The "Niplette": an instrument for the non-surgical correction of inverted nipples [see comments]. *British Journal of Plastic Surgery*. 1994 Jan; **47(1)**:46–9. [Table 16]

McIntosh J. Barriers to breastfeeding; Choice of feeding method in a sample of working class primipari. *Midwifery*. 1985; **1**:213–224.

McLachlan Z, Milne E J, Lumley J, & Walker B L. Ultrasound treatment for breast engorgement: a randomised double blind trial. *Australian Journal of Physiotherapy*. 1991; **37**:23–29. [Table 74]

McNeilly A. The physiology of lactation. *Journal of Biosocial Science*. 1977; Supplement **4**:5–21.

Miller J J, McVeagh P, Fleet G H, Petocz P, & Brand J C. Breath hydrogen excretion in infants with colic. *Archives of Disease in Childhood*. 1989; **64**:725–729.

Miller S A, & Chopra J G. Problems with Human Milk and Infant Formulas. *Pediatrics*. 1984; Supplement **74(2)**:639–647.

Milsom S R, Breier B H, Gallaher B W, Cox V A, Gunn A J, & Gluckman P

D. Growth hormone stimulates galactopoiesis in healthy lactating women. *Acta Endocrinologica*. 1992; **127**:337–343. [Table 110]

Minchin M. Breastfeeding matters. Alma Publications; 1998.

Ministry of Agriculture, Fisheries and Food. The British Diet: Finding the Facts. *Food Surveillance Paper.* HMSO. 1994.

Mitchell E A, Taylor B J, Ford R P, Stewart A W, Becroft D M, Thompson J M, Scragg R, Hassal I B, Barry D M, Allen E M et al. Dummies and the sudden infant death syndrome. *Archives of Disease in Childhood*. 1993; **68(4)**:501–4.

Moore D J, Robb T A, & Davidson G P. Breath hydrogen response to milk containing lactose in colicky and non-colicky infants. *Journal of Pediatrics*. 1988; **113(6)**:979–984.

Morse J M, Ewing G, Gamble D, and Donahue P. The effect of maternal fluid intake on breast milk supply: a pilot study. *Canadian Journal of Public Health/Revue Canadienne de Sante Publique*. 1992 May; **83(3)**:213–6. [Table 91]

Morse J M, Jehle C, & Gamble D. Initiating breastfeeding: a world survey of the timing of postpartum breastfeeding. *International Journal of Nursing Studies*. 1990; **27(3)**:303–13. [Table 17]

Murata T, Hunzow M, and Nomura Y. The clinical effects of 'Protease complex' on postpartum breast engorgement. *Journal of Japanese Obstetric Gynaecological Society*. 1965; **12(3)**:139–147. [Table 78]

Myles M F. Textbook for Midwives. Eighth ed. Edinburgh: Churchill Livingstone; 1975.

National Childbirth Trust. Hypoglycaemia of the Newborn. London: NCT Maternity Sales; 1997. ISBN: 1 870129 96 2.

Neifert M R. Infant problems in breast-feeding. In "Lactation: Physiology, Nutrition, and Breast-feeding." Eds. M C Neville & M R Neifert, Plenum Press, 1983; Chap 4, pp 303–32.

Neifert M, Lawrence R, & Seacat J. Nipple confusion: toward a formal definition. *Journal of Pediatrics*. 1995; **126(6)**:S125–9.

Neifert M, Gray J, Gary N, & Camp B. Effect of two types of hospital feeding gift packs on duration of breastfeeding among adolescent mothers. *Journal of Adolescent Health Care*. 1988; **9**:41–3. [Table 65]

Neifert M, de Marzo S, Seacat J, Young D, Leff M, and Orleans M. The influence of breast surgery, breast appearance, and pregnancy-induced breast changes on lactation sufficiency as measured by infant weight gain. *Birth*. 1990; **17(1)**:31–8. [Table 89]

Neifert M R, & Seacat J M. Lactation insufficiency: a rational approach. *Birth*. 1987; **14**:182–188.

Newton M, & Newton N R. The letdown reflex in human lactation. *Journal of Pediatrics*. 1948; **33**:698–704.

Nicholson W L. Cracked nipples in breastfeeding mothers. *Journal of the Nursing Mothers Association of Australia*. 1985; **21(4)**:7–10. [Table 68]

Nicholson W L. The use of nipple shields by breastfeeding women. *Journal of the Australian College of Midwives*. 1993; **6(2)**:18–24. [Table 69]

Nicoll A, Ginsburg R, and Tripp J H. Supplementary feeding and jaundice in newborns. *Acta Paediatrica Scandinavica*. 1982; **71(5)**:759–61. [Table 45]

Nikodem V C, Danziger D, Gebka N, Gulmezoglu A M, and Hofmeyr G J. Do cabbage leaves prevent breast engorgement? A randomized, controlled study. *Birth*. 1993; **20(2)**:61–4. [Table 75]

Notestine G E. The importance of the identification of ankyloglossia (short lingual frenulum) as a cause of breastfeeding problems. *Journal of Human Lactation*. 1990; **6(3)**:113–5. [Table 121]

Nylander G, Lindemann R, Helsing E, & Bendvold E. Unsupplemented breastfeeding in the maternity ward: positive long-term effects. *Acta Obstet. Gynecol. Scand.* 1991; **70**:205–9. [Table 49]

Ogaard B, Larsson E, & Lindsten R. The effect of sucking habits, cohort, sex, intercanine arch widths, and breast or bottle feeding on posterior crossbite in Norwegian and Swedish 3-year-old children. *American Journal or Orthodontics & Dentofacial Orthopedics*. 1994; **106(2)**:161–6.

Olmstead R W, & Jackson E B. Self-demand feeding in the first week of life. *Pediatrics*. 1950; **6**:396–401.

Palmer G. The Politics of breastfeeding. London: Pandora; 1993.

Peaker M, and Wilde C J. Evidence for local feedback control of human milk secretion. *News in Physiological Science*. 1987; **2**:124–6.

Peaker M, and Wilde C J. Autocrine regulation of milk secretion by a protein in milk. *Biochemical Journal*. 1995; **305**:51–8.

Perez-Escamilla R, Roman Perez R, Mejia L A, & Dewey K G. Infant feeding practices among low-income Mexican urban women: a four month follow-up. *Archivos Latinoamericanos De Nutricion*. 1992; **42(3)**:259–67.

Perez-Escamilla R, Pollitt E, Lonnerdal B, & Dewey KG. Infant feeding policies on maternity wards and their effect on breast-feeding success: an analytical overview. *American Journal of Public Health*. 1994, **84(1)**:89–97.

Peters F, Schulze-Tollert J, & Schuth W. Thyrotrophin-releasing hormone – a lactation-promoting agent?. *British Journal of Obstetrics & Gynaecology*. 1991; **98(9)**:880–5. [Table 108]

Petraglia F, de Leo V, Sardelli S, Pieroni M L, d'Antona N, & Genazzani A R. Domperidone in defective and insufficient lactation. *European Journal of Obstetrics, Gynecology, & Reproductive Biology*. 1985; **19(5)**:281–7. [Table 105]

Prasad B, & Costello A M. Impact and sustainability of a "baby friendly" health education intervention at a district hospital in Bihar, India. *British Medical Journal*. 1995; **310(6980)**:621–623. [Table 26]

Pugh L C, Buchko B L, Bishop B A, Cochran J F, Smith L R, & Lerew D J. A comparison of topical agents to relieve nipple pain and enhance breastfeeding. *Birth*. 1996; **23(2)**:88–93. [Table 37]

Pugin E, Valdés V, Labbok M H, Pérez A, & Aravena R. Does prenatal breastfeeding skills group education increase the effectiveness of a comprehensive breastfeeding promotion program? *Journal of Human Lactation.* 1996; **12(1)**:15–19.

Read L C, Tarantal A S George-Nascimenti C. Effects of recombinant human epidermal growth factor on the intestinal growth of fetal rhesus monkeys. *Acta Paediatrica Scandinavica.* 1988; **351(Suppl.)**:97–103.

Reyntjens A J, Niemegeers C J E, Van Neuten J M, and Laduron P. Domperidone: a novel and safe gastrokinetic antinauseant for the treatment of dyspepsia and vomiting. *Arzneimittelforschung.* 1978; **28**:1194–1196.

Rickitt C W. A study in nipple care. *Midwives Chronicle.* 1986; **99(1181)**:131–2. [Table 34]

Righard L. Are breastfeeding problems related to incorrect breastfeeding technique and the use of pacifiers and bottles? *Birth.* 1998; **25(1)**:40–44. [Table 56]

Righard L, & Alade M O. Effect of delivery room routines on success of first breast-feed. *The Lancet.* 1990; **336(8723)**:1105–7. [Table 25]

Righard L, & Alade M O. Sucking technique and its effect on success of breastfeeding. *Birth.* 1992; **19(4)**:185–9. [Table 30]

Righard L, & Alade M O. Breastfeeding and the use of pacifiers. *Birth.* 1997; **24(2)**:116–20.

Righard L, Flodmark C-E, Lothe L, & Jakobsson I. Breastfeeding patterns: comparing the effects on infant behavior and maternal satisfaction of using one or two breasts. *Birth.* 1993; **20(4)**:182–5. [Table 116]

Riordan J. The effectiveness of topical agents in reducing nipple soreness of breastfeeding mothers. *Journal of Human Lactation.* 1985; **1(3)**:36–41. [Table 35]

Riordan J M, & Nichols F H. A descriptive study of lactation mastitis in long-term breastfeeding women. *Journal of Human Lactation.* 1990; **6(2)**:53–8. [Table 82]

Riordan J, & Auerbach K G. Breastfeeding and human lactation. Boston: Jones and Bartlett Publishers; 1993.

Roberts K L. A comparison of chilled cabbage leaves and chilled gelpacks in reducing breast engorgement. *Journal of Human Lactation.* 1995a; **11(1)**:17–20. [Table 76]

Roberts K L, Reiter M, and Schuster D. A comparison of chilled and room temperature cabbage leaves in treating breast engorgement. *Journal of Human Lactation.* 1995b; **11(3)**:191–4. [Table 77]

Rosenberg M. Breast-Feeding and Infant Mortality in Norway 1860–1930. *Journal of Biosocial Science.* 1989; **21**:335–348.

Rosenblatt K A, & Thomas D B. WHO Collaborative study of neoplasia and steroid contraceptives. *International Journal of Epidemiology.* 1993, **22**:192–7.

Royal College of Midwives. Successful Breastfeeding: A practical guide for midwives. Edinburgh: Churchill Livingstone; 1991 2nd Edtn.

Saarinen U M, & Kajosaari M. Breastfeeding as prophylaxis against atopic disease: prospective follow-up study until 17 years old. *Lancet.* 1995; **346(8982)**:1065–9.

Sachdev H P S, Krishna J, Puri R K, Satyanarayana L & Kumar S. Water supplementation in exclusively breastfed infants during summer in the tropics. *The Lancet.* 1991; **337(8747)**:929–33.

Saint L, Smith M, and Hartman P E. The yield and nutrient content of colostrum and milk of women giving birth to one month postpartum. *British Journal of Nutrition.* 1984; **52**:87–95.

Sakashita R, Kamegai T, & Inoue N. Masseter muscle activity in bottle feeding with the chewing type bottle teat: evidence from electromyographs. *Early Human Development.* 1996; **45**:83–92.

Salariya E M, Easton P M, and Cater J I. Duration of breast-feeding after early initiation and frequent feeding. *Lancet.* 1978 Nov 25; **2(8100)**:1141–3. [Table 21]

Schubiger G, Schwarz U & Tönz O. UNICEF/WHO Baby-Friendly Hospital Initiative: Does the use of bottles and pacifiers in the neonatal nursery prevent successful breastfeeding? *European Journal of Pediatrics.* 1997; **156**:874–7. [Table 55]

Sharma S, Ramji S Kumari S & Bapna J S. Randomized controlled trial of Asparagus racemosus (Shatavari) as a lactogogue in lactational inadequacy. *Indian Pediatrics.* 1996; **33**:675–7. [Table 112]

Sharp D. Moist wound healing for cracked nipples. *Breastfeeding Abstracts.* 1992; **12(2)**:19.

Sikorski J, Renfrew M J. Support for breastfeeding mothers. The Cochrane Library 1999; Issue 3. Update Software, Oxford, UK.

Silb J A, & Glass E J. Metoclopramide in young children. *British Medical Journal.* 1978; **2**:431.

Simsarian F P, & McLendon P A. Feeding behaviour of an infant during the first twelve weeks of life on a self-demand schedule. *Journal of Pediatrics.* 1942; **20**:93–103.

Slaven S, Craft I and Harvey D R. A double-blind controlled trial of chlorhexidine in aerosol spray for the prevention of sore nipples. Unpublished. 1988. [Table 32]

Smith B A M. Feeding overstrength cow's milk to babies. *British Medical Journal.* 1974; **iv**: 741–2.

Smith W L. Erenburg A, Nowak A & Franken E A. Physiology of sucking in the normal term infant using real-time ultrasound. *Radiology.* 1985; **156**:379–81.

Snell B J, Krantz M, Keeton R, Delgado K, & Peckham C. The association of formula samples given at hospital discharge with the early duration of breastfeeding. *Journal of Human Lactation.* 1992; **8(2)**:67–72. [Table 62]

Spangler A, & Hildebrandt E. The effect of modified lanolin on nipple pain/damage during the first ten days of breastfeeding. *International Journal of Childbirth Education.* 1993 Aug; **8(3)**:15–9.

Standing Committee on Nutrition of the British Paediatric Association. "Is breast feeding beneficial in the UK?". *Archives of Disease in Childhood.* 1994; **71**:376–380.

Storr G B. Prevention of nipple tenderness and breast engorgement in the postpartal period. *JOGNN – Journal of Obstetric, Gynecologic, & Neonatal Nursing.* 1988 May; **17(3)**:203–9. [Table 6]

Taitz L S, & Byers H D. High calorie/osmolar feeding and hypertonic dehydration. *Archives of Disease in Childhood.* 1972; **47**:257–60.

Tanguay K E, McBean M R, and Jain E. Nipple candidiasis among breastfeeding mothers. Case-control study of predisposing factors. *Canadian Family Physician* 1994 Aug; **40**:1407–13.

Taubman B. Curing Infant Colic. New York: Bantam Books; 1990.

Taylor P M, Taylor F H, Campbell S B, Maloni J A, and Cannon M. Extra early physical contact and aspects of the mother-infant relationship. *Acta Paediatrica Scandinavica.* 1985; **1416**:3–14.

Terrill P J, & Stapleton M J. The inverted nipple: to cut the ducts or not?. *British Journal of Plastic Surgery.* 1991 Jul; **44(5)**:372–7. [Table 14]

Thomsen A C, Espersen T, and Maigaard S. Course and treatment of milk stasis, non-infectious inflammation of the breast, and infectious mastitis in nursing women. *American Journal of Obstetrics & Gynecology.* 1984 Jul 1; **149(5)**:492–5. [Table 86]

Uhari M, Mantysaari K, & Niemala M. A meta-analytic review of the risk factors for acute otitis media. *Clinical Infectious Disease.* 1996; **22(6)**:1079–83.

United Kingdom National Case-Control Study Group. Breastfeeding and risk of breast cancer in young women. *British Medical Journal.* 1993; **307**:17–20.

Valdés V, Pérez A, Labbok M, Pugin E, Zambrano I, and Catalan S. The impact of a hospital and clinic-based breastfeeding promotion programme in a middle class urban environment. *Journal of Tropical Pediatrics.* 1993 Jun; **39(3)**:142–51. [Table 24]

Verronen P. Breastfeeding: reasons for giving up and transient lactational crisis. *Acta Paediatrica Scandinavica.* 1982; **71**:447–450.

Victora C G, Tomasi E, Olinto M T, & Barros F C. Use of pacifiers and breastfeeding duration. *The Lancet.* 1993; **341(8842)**:404–6.

Victora C G, Behague D P, Barros F C, Olinto M T, & Weiderpass E. Pacifier use and short breastfeeding duration: cause, consequence or coincidence? *Pediatrics.* 1997; **99(3)**:445–53.

Waldenstrom U, & Nilsson C A. No effect of birth centre care on either duration or experience of breast feeding, but more complications: findings from a randomised controlled trial. *Midwifery.* 1994 Mar; **10(1)**:8–17.

Walker M. A fresh look at the risks of artificial infant feeding. *Journal of Human Lactation.* 1993 Jun; **9(2)**:97–107.

Walker M, & Auerbach K G. Breast pumps and other technologies. In "Breastfeeding and Human Lactation", Eds J Riordan & K G Auerbach. Chapter 11, pp 279–332. Jones and Bartlett, Boston. 1993.

Waller H. The early failure of breastfeeding. *Archives of Disease in Childhood.* 1946; **21**:1–12. [Table 1]

Watase S, Mourine A P, & Tipton G A. An analysis of malocclusion in children with otitis media. *Pediatric Dentistry.* 1998; **20(5)**:327–30.

Weatherley-White R C, Kuehn D P, Mirrett P, Gilman J I, and Weatherley-White C C. Early repair and breast-feeding for infants with cleft lip. *Plastic & Reconstructive Surgery.* 1987 Jun; **79(6)**:879–885. [Table 118]

Weber F, Woolridge M W, and Baum J D. An ultrasonographic study of the organisation of sucking and swallowing by newborn infants. *Developmental Medicine & Child Neurology.* 1986; **28**:19–24.

White A, Freeth S, and O'Brien M. Infant feeding 1990: survey carried out for the DHSS by the Office of Population Censuses and Surveys. London: Her Majesty's Stationery Office; 1992.

Whitley N. Preparation for breastfeeding. *Journal of Obstetric, Gynaecologic, and Neonatal Nursing.* 1978; **7**:44–48. [Table 10]

Widstrom A M, Ransjo-Arvidson A B, Christensson K, Matthiesen A S, Winberg J, and Uvnas-Moberg K. Gastric suction in healthy newborn infants. Effects on circulation and developing feeding behaviour. *Acta Paediatrica Scandinavica.* 1987 Jul; **76(4)**:566–72. [Table 28]

Widstrom A M, Wahlberg V, Matthiesen A S, Eneroth P, Uvnas-Moberg K, Werner S, and Winberg J. Short-term effects of early suckling and touch of the nipple on maternal behaviour. *Early Human Development.* 1990 Mar; **21(3)**:153–63. [Table 19]

Wilde C J, Addey C V P and Peaker M. Feedback control of milk secretion from milk. *Journal of Mammary Gland Biology & Neoplasia.* 1995; **1**:307–15.

Williams A. Hypoglycaemia of the newborn: a review. *Bulletin of the World Health Organization.* 1997; **75(3)**:261–90.

Willis C E, & Livingstone V. Infant insufficient milk syndrome associated with maternal postpartum hemorrhage. *Journal of Human Lactation.* 1995 Jun; **11(2)**:123–6. [Table 87]

Wilson A C, Forsyth J S, Greene S S, Irvine I, Hau C, & Howie P W. Relation of infant diet to childhood health: seven year follow up of cohort of children in Dundee infant feeding study. *British Medical Journal.* 1998; **316**:21–5.

Winberg J, & de Chateau P. Attempts to increase breast-feeding. Proceeding 5th Intl Congress Psychosomatic Obstet & Gynaecol, Rome 1979. In "Emotion and Reproduction" pp 851–4.

Woessner C, Lauwers J & Bernard B. Breastfeeding Today: A Mother's Companion. New York: Avery Publishing Group Inc, 1987.

Woolridge M W. The 'anatomy' of infant sucking. *Midwifery.* 1986a; **2(4)**:164–71.

Woolridge M W. Aetiology of sore nipples. *Midwifery.* 1986b; **2(4)**:172–6.

Woolridge M W. Baby-controlled breastfeeding: biocultural implications. P Stuart-Macadam & K A Dettwyler (Eds). Breastfeeding: Biocultural Perspectives. New York: Aldine De Gruyter; 1995; pp. 217–242.

Woolridge M W. "Breastfeeding: physiology into practice." In *Nutrition in Child Health.* Ed D P Davies. Proceedings of conference jointly organised by the Royal College of Physicians of London and the British Paediatric Association. RCPL Press; 1995; pp. 13–31.

Woolridge M W. Problems of establishing lactation. *Food and Nutrition Bulletin.* 1996; **17(4)**:316–323.

Woolridge M W, Baum J D, and Drewett R F. Does a change in the composition of human milk affect sucking patterns and intake. *The Lancet.* 1980a; **2(8207)**:1292–1293.

Woolridge M W, Baum J D, and Drewett R F. Effect of a traditional and of a new nipple shield on sucking patterns and milk flow. *Early Human Development.* 1980b; **4(4)**:357–64. [Table 66]

Woolridge M W, Baum J D, and Drewett R F. Individual patterns of milk intake during breast-feeding. *Early Human Development.* 1982; **7(3)**:265–72. [Table 44]

Woolridge M W, Greasley V, & Silpisornkosol S. The initiation of lactation: the effect of early versus delayed contact for suckling on milk intake in the first week post-partum. A study in Chiang Mai, Northern Thailand. *Early Human Development.* 1985; **12**:269–78. [Table 22]

Woolridge M W, & Fisher C. Colic 'overfeeding' and symptoms of lactose malabsorption in the breastfed baby: a possible artifact of feeding management? *The Lancet.* 1988 **ii**: 382–384.

WHO/UNICEF Joint Meeting on Infant and Young Child Feeding, Geneva, 9th–12th October 1979; ratified by resolution 33.32 of the World Health Assembly. May 1980.

World Health Organization. Contemporary patterns of breast-feeding: Report on the WHO Collaborative Study on Breast-feeding. W.H.O. Geneva: 1981. 211 pp. [citation from Chapter 4, pp 31–46]

World Health Organization, & UNICEF. Protecting, promoting and supporting breast-feeding: the special role of maternity services. Geneva: 1989.

World Health Organization. The World Health Organization's infant feeding recommendation. *Weekly epidemiological record.* 1995, **70**:119–120.

World Health Organization. Evidence for the ten steps to successful breastfeeding. WHO Geneva: 1998. WHO/CHD/98.9

Wright A L, Holberg C J, Martinez F D, Morgan W J, Taussig L M. Breastfeeding and lower respiratory tract illness in the first year of life. *British Medical Journal.* 1989; **299**:946–9.

Yamauchi Y, & Yamanouchi I. The relationship between rooming-in/not rooming-in and breast-feeding variables. *Acta Paediatrica Scandinavica.*

1990 Nov; **79(11)**:1017–22.

Ylikorkala O, Kauppila A, Kivinen S, and Viinikka L. Sulpiride improves inadequate lactation. *British Medical Journal*. 1982; **285**:249–251. [Table 103]

Ylikorkala O, Kauppila A, Kivinen S, and Viinikka L. Treatment of inadequate lactation with oral sulpiride and buccal oxytocin. *Obstetrics & Gynecology*. 1984 Jan; **63(1)**:57–60. [Table 104]

Ylikorkala O, Kivinen S, and Kauppila A. Oral administration of TRH in puerperal women: effect on insufficient lactation, thyroid hormones and on the responses of TSH and prolactin to intravenous TRH. *Acta Endocrinologica*. 1980 Apr; **93(4)**:413–8. [Table 107]

Zarate A, Villalobos H, Canales E, Soria J, Arcovedo F, and MacGregor C. The effect of oral administration of thyrotrophin-releasing hormone on lactation. *Journal of Clinical Endocrinology and Metabolism*. 1976; **43**:301–305. [Tables 109a & b]

Ziemer M M, Cooper D M, & Pigeon J G. Evaluation of a dressing to reduce nipple pain and improve nipple skin condition in breastfeeding women. *Nursing Research*. 1995; **44(6)**:347–51. [Table 71]

Appendices

I. **Search Strategy**
   Bibliography of support, advice and information

II. **Tables – 1–121**

APPENDIX I

Details of search strategy

Sources searched

The following electronic databases were searched:

Cochrane Pregnancy and Childbirth Database (up to and including 1997 Issue 4)

MEDLINE 1966-1997

Bath Information and Data Services (BIDS) 1985-1997

Cumulative Index of Nursing Research and the Allied Literature (CINAHL) 1983-1997

The Midwifery Research Database (MIRIAD) 1988-1997

Midwives Information and Resource Service database (MIDIRS) 1985-1997

Health Service Management Information Service (HELMIS)

In addition, the following sources were searched by hand:

The Journal of Human Lactation 1985-1997

Reference lists from:

Inch S Antenatal preparation for breastfeeding

Inch S and Garforth S Establishing and maintaining breastfeeding

Inch S and Renfrew MJ Common breastfeeding problems
    all in Chalmers I, Enkin M and Keirse MJNC (eds) 'Effective Care in Pregnancy and Childbirth' 1989. Oxford University Press, Oxford.

Lawrence RA. Breastfeeding, a guide for the medical profession (4th edition). 1994. Mosby, St Louis

Riordan J and Auerbach KG. Breastfeeding and Human Lactation. 1993. Jones and Bartlett, Boston and London.

Terms used for computer-based searches

\#

1. exp breast feeding/
2. exp lactation disorders/
3. milk, human/
4. (breastfeed$ or breast-feed$ or breastfeed$).tw.
5. nipples/
6. ((sore or cracked or size or inverted or flat) adj nipple$).tw.
7. exp maternal-child nursing/
8. ((insufficient or poor or absence or lack or failure) adj2 milk).tw.
9. feeding difficulties.tw.
10. (baby or babies).tw.
11. 9 and 10
12. exp infant, newborn, diseases/
13. ((engorge$ or infection$ or abscess) adj2 breast$).tw.
14. drug therapy/
15. ointments/
16. (position$ and (breastfeeding or breast feeding or breast-feeding)).tw.
17. surgery/
18. (nipple shield$ or breast pump$ or hand express$).tw.
19. nipple shield$.tw.
20. 18 or 19
21. exp alternative medicine/
22. breast feeding.tw.
23. 1 or 3 or 4 or 22
24. 2 or 5 or 6 or 8 or 11 or 12 or 13
25. 7 or 23
26. 14 or 15 or 16 or 17 or 18 or 19 or 21
27. 24 and 25 and 26
28. lactation disorders/dt,pc,th
29. 27 or 28
30. 24 and 25
31. limit 30 to English language
32. limit 31 to human
33. limit 29 to English language
34. limit 33 to human

This search strategy was used initially for searching up to the end of 1996.

An amended version was then used to search for publications in 1997 and to re-check journals up to and including 1996. Additional lines were included to search for trials and experimental studies (as set out for Cochrane Reviews).

#
1. exp breast feeding/
2. milk, human/
3. (breastfeed$ or breast-feed$ or (breast adj feed$)).tw.
4. or/1-3
5. exp lactation disorders/
6. nipples/
7. ((sore or crack$ or fissure$ or size or small or large adj2 nipple$).tw.
8. (flat or invert$ or retract$ or prtract$ or non-protract$) adj2 nipple|$))
9. ((insufficient or poor or absence or lack or failure) adj2 (milk or supply)).tw.
10. (breast$ adj2 (engorge$ or infection$ or absces$ or abces$)).tw.
11 (position$ and (breastfeeding or breast-feeding or (breast adj feeding))).tw.
12. (nipple adj2 shield$) or (breast adj2 pump$) or (hand adj2 express$).tw.
13. or/5-12
14. exp maternal-child nursing/
15. exp infant, newborn, diseases/
16. feeding difficulties.tw.
17. 14 and 16
18 (baby or babies or infant or newborn).tw.
19. 16 and 18
20. (poor or slow or inadequate) adj2 (weight or gain)).tw.
21 17 or 19 or 20
22. drug therapy/
23. ointments/
24. surgery/
25. or/22-24
26. 13 or 21 or 25
27. 4 and 26
28. limit 27 to English language
29. limit 28 to human
30. clinical trials/
31. randomized controlled trials/
32. random allocation/
33. double-blind method/
34. single blind method/
35. (blind adj2 (method$ or study or comparison$)).tw.
36. ((random$ or control$) adj2 (trial$ or study or allocat$)).tw.
37. or/30-36
38. 4 and 37
39. 26 and 37
40. limit 38 to English language
41. limit 40 to human
42. limit 39 to English language
43. limit 42 to human

APPENDIX II
Tables

TABLE 1: The early failure of breast feeding

Method: Non-randomised prospective comparison study

Authors	Date	Where published	Intervention assessed	Entry criteria	Number of women studied	Outcomes measured	Results
Waller H	1946	Arch Dis Child 21: 1–12	Antenatal expression of colostrum versus No antenatal expression Expression commenced up to 3 months before delivery	Lactating women	200 100 in control group 100 in treatment group	Duration of breastfeeding: Fully breastfeeding on discharge Fully breastfeeding at 3 months Fully breastfeeding at 6 months Incidence of breast complications	97/100 of the treatment group were fully breastfeeding compared with 83/100 of the control group 87/100 of the treatment group were breastfeeding at 3 months compared with 65/100 of the controls At 6 months 83 of the treatment group were breastfeeding in comparison to 42 of the controls Significantly less engorgement and damaged nipples in the treatment group

TABLE 2: Breast-feeding: factors affecting success

Method: Non-randomised prospective comparison study

Authors	Date	Where published	Intervention assessed	Entry criteria	Number of women studied	Outcomes measured	Results
Blaikeley J Clarke S Mackeith R Ogden KM	1953	J Obstet Gynaecol Br Emp 60: 657–669	Antenatal expression of colostrum (This treatment began daily 4 to 8 weeks before delivery) versus No treatment	Primiparous women who lived within 3 miles of the hospital; delivered in the ward of the hospital	234 117 in treatment group 117 in control group	Duration of breastfeeding Fully breastfeeding at discharge Fully breastfeeding at 3 months Fully breastfeeding at 6 months Incidence of breast complications	102/117 of the treatment group 97/117 of the control group 76/117 in the treatment group 60/117 in the control group 56/117 in the treatment group 40/117 in the control group Significantly less engorgement and damaged nipples in the treatment group

TABLE 3: The value of antenatal massage of nipples and expression of colostrum

Method: Non-randomised cohort comparison study

Authors	Date	Where published	Intervention assessed	Entry criteria	Number of women studied	Outcomes measured	Results
Ingelman-Sundberg A	1958	J Obstet Gynaecol Br Empire 65: 448–449	Instruction in antenatal breast massage and expression of colostrum from 20th week of pregnancy versus No treatment	The experimental group were the patients of the author The control group were the patients of his 2 colleagues Postnatally mothers having preterm infants were excluded from the investigation	Experimental group = 313 Control group = 343	Fully breastfeeding at time of discharge Total amount of milk suckled and expressed on the 7th day after delivery Frequency of mastitis during stay in hospital	Experimental group = 94% fully breastfeeding Control group = 93% fully breastfeeding Experimental group = 417 ± 151g Control group = 399 ± 131 g Experimental group = 2.88% ±0.95 Control group = 0.88% ±0.51

TABLE 4: Preparation of the breast for breastfeeding

Method: A randomised trial

Authors	Date	Where published	Intervention assessed	Entry criteria	Number of women studied	Outcomes measured	Results
Brown MS Hurlock JT	1975	Nursing Research 24(6): 448–451	3 weeks before the expected date of their delivery, each of the women were randomly assigned to one of the three groups 1. Nipple rolling 2. Application of Masse cream 3. Expression of colostrum The women carried out one of these methods twice a day on one nipple only	Not breastfed previously, and if any mother and baby pair had an extended hospital stay because of complications, their data were discarded	57	Nipple pain	There was no table of results but in the discussion it mentioned that there was no significant difference between groups

TABLE 5: A comparison of the effectiveness of two methods of nipple care

Method: Non-randomised prospective comparison study

Authors	Date	Where published	Intervention assessed	Entry criteria	Number of women studied	Outcomes measured	Results
Hewat RJ Ellis DJ	1987	Birth 14(1): 41–5	Comparison between the effectiveness of the application of expressed breastmilk: a. with that of hydrous lanolin b. to women's nipples following breastfeeding Women were their own control using: a. on one breast and b. on the other	No known allergy to wool Lived within 10 miles of the hospital	23	Nipple pain perceived by the women. Nipple trauma was assessed on postpartum day 0, 1, 2, 3, 5, 7, and 10	Nipple pain perceived by the women was similar in both groups, as was nipple trauma 95% of the women experienced nipple pain, and postpartum day 3 was when nipple pain was most intense

TABLE 6: Prevention of nipple tenderness and breast engorgement in the postpartal period

Method: Non-randomised prospective comparison study

Authors	Date	Where published	Intervention assessed	Entry criteria	Number of women studied	Outcomes measured	Results
Storr GB	1988	J Obstet Gynaecol Neontl Med 17(3): 203–209	Preparing one nipple and massaging one breast Nipple rolling twice daily for 30 seconds Rub nipple gently with terry towel for 15 seconds twice daily	Volunteers recruited from a group of women attending prenatal programme	25 Own controls	Does prenatal nipple conditioning influence nipple tenderness? Does prophylactic postpartal breast massage decrease the incidence of engorgement?	Significantly less tenderness with prepared breast (p=0.001) Significantly less overall engorgement with prepared breast (p=0.004)

TABLE 7: Prenatal nipple conditioning for breastfeeding

Method: Non-randomised prospective comparison study

Authors	Date	Where published	Intervention assessed	Entry criteria	Number of women studied	Outcomes measured	Results
Atkinson LD	1979	Nursing Research 28(5): 267–271	Prenatal nipple conditioning began 6 weeks before breastfeeding was due to start. Conditioned one nipple only and the other nipple acted as the control. Conditioning consisted of: 1. Gentle nipple rubbing with a terry towel for 15 seconds. 2. Nipple rolling twice a day for 2 minutes 3. Airing the nipple for 2 hours a day, leaving it exposed and allowing the outer clothes to rub against the nipple	Primigravida, planned to breastfeed, did not have inverted nipples, right handed.	22 women enlisted 17 completed study	Nipple pain in the first 5 days after delivery	6 women reported no difference in nipple pain between the conditioned nipple and the unconditioned nipple 11 women reported significantly less extreme pain in the nipple that had been conditioned *Based on 477 observations for all 17 women summed across five days*
						Effect of skin tone on nipple pain	7 women with fair skin reported slightly higher rates of extreme pain than the 7 women with average skin type or the 3 women with olive skin *The numbers of women in the study are too small to draw any valid conclusions*

TABLE 8: The effect of prenatal nipple conditioning on postpartum nipple pain in breastfeeding women

Method: Prospective within-subject trial

Authors	Date	Where published	Intervention assessed	Entry criteria	Number of women studied	Outcomes measured	Results
Fleming PA	1984	Health Care for Women Intl 5: 453–7	Antenatal nipple conditioning of one nipple, the other acting as control. Conditioning comprised gentle rubbing of the nipples with a towel (15sec/day), nipple rolling (2min/day) and nipple exposure to allow them to rub against outer clothing (2hr/day). *NB Partial replication of study by Atkinson [Table 7]*	Women attending childbirth preparation classes	17 women enrolled 14 completed study (data from all 17 women analysed)	Nipple pain rated on a 3-point scale	Women had more ratings of 'negligible' pain (p<0.025), and fewer ratings of 'definite' (not significant) and 'extreme' pain (p<0.01) on the conditioned nipple, compared to the unconditioned nipple *These comparisons were based on cumulative frequencies of observations (n=259) from the same women, pain ratings being summed for every breastfeed across all days spent in hospital; this invalidates the statistical comparison*

TABLE 9: A study of four methods of nipple care offered to postpartum mothers

Method: Non-randomised prospective comparison study

Authors	Date	Where published	Intervention assessed	Entry criteria	Number of women studied	Outcomes measured	Results
Clark M	1985	The New Zealand Nursing Journal 16–18	Four different methods of nipple care were assessed, each over a separate period of 30 days In addition women were also asked if they had performed any antenatal nipple preparation 1. Routine care: mothers were given advice and assistance with positioning; heat via sunshine or heat lamp was used to relieve nipple pain; nipple shield was offered for severe pain. Cream or ointment was used as desired by the mothers. Infants were fed 3- or 4-hourly for the first 48 hours and then on demand	Breastfeeding mothers who were admitted to the postnatal ward soon after delivery and who consented to participation	114	Nipple pain at 4 days postpartum The difference in nipple pain between mothers who had carried out some method of antenatal nipple preparation and those who had not (type of method not discussed)	90% of mothers complained of nipple pain 9.8% were pain free The highest number of cracked nipples occured in the group undertaking antenatal preparation (36% versus 19%), although the number reporting nipple tenderness was proportionately less in that group (64% versus 81%)

TABLE 9: *continued*

Authors	Date	Where published	Intervention assessed	Entry criteria	Number of women studied	Outcomes measured	Results
			2. Heat: Same treatment as used in routine care but no creams or ointments were offered 3. Heat lamp: Used after feeding approximately 3 times daily 4. Vitamin A: The same routine care but the only ointment used was Vitamin A cream used after each feed 5. Anhydrous lanolin: The same routine care, anhydrous lanolin used as the ointment, this was used after each feed			Comparison of nipple pain, cracked nipples, and number of women discontinuing breastfeeding between the four methods of nipple care	The greatest number of cracked nipples occurred in the heat only group, 46% compared with a mean of 25% in the other three groups In the heat only group 15.3% discontinued feeding compared with a mean of 5% in the other groups The group using anhydrous lanolin were more likely to be discharged symptom free than the other groups. 96.5% did not have painful nipples at discharge compared with 57.1% in the routine care group, 69.2% in the group treated with heat and 78.5% in the group treated with Vitamin A ointment

TABLE 10: Preparation for breastfeeding

Method: Retrospective survey

Authors	Date	Where published	Method	Purpose	Results
Whitley N	1978	JOGNN 7: 44–48	Telephone interviews with 68-item questionnaire The interview took between 30–45 minutes	A follow up survey, at one year after delivery, of breastfeeding mothers who had had either conventional antenatal or Lamaze classes The purpose of the study was to determine the type of breastfeeding experience these women had, what effect the antenatal classes had, and how long they had breastfed	Data was collected on 34 women, 22 were primiparas and 12 multiparas. The duration of breastfeeding was divided into three groups: Group 1. Fed for less than 6 weeks = 6 (18%) Group 2. Fed for 6–23 weeks = 11 (32%) Group 3. Fed for 24 or more weeks = 17 (50%) Breast massage and hand expression of colostrum had been taught, and 28 women practiced this. The results of the survey indicated that there was almost no difference in the incidence of engorgement, nor in the duration of breastfeeding Nipple rolling during pregnancy did not appear to prevent sore nipples. 24 of the women carried out nipple rolling, 16 (67%) developed sore nipples, 10 women did not practice this and only 5 (50%) developed sore nipples Women who had restricted nursing times were significantly more likely to report nipple pain than those who practiced flexible feeding patterns

TABLE 11: Pain or pleasure: The dilemma of early breastfeeding

Method: Prospective cohort study (survey)

Authors	Date	Where published	Intervention assessed	Entry criteria	Number of women studied	Outcomes measured	Results
L'Esperance CM	1980	Birth and the Family Journal 7(1): 21–26	1. Women were interviewed in the first 24 hours after delivery, regarding their previous breastfeeding experience; details of any nipple conditioning antenatally 2. Women were asked to record nipple pain and degree of engorgement at 48 hours, 72 hours and 96 hours after delivery	No mention of entry criteria	120	Factors related to nipple discomfort	Antenatal nipple conditioning had no significant effect on postpartum nipple pain Engorgement of the breast increased nipple pain

TABLE 12: Randomised controlled trial of breast shells and Hoffman's exercises for inverted and non-protractile nipples

Method: Randomised controlled trial

Authors	Date	Where published	Intervention assessed	Entry criteria	Number of women studied	Outcomes measured	Results
Alexander JM Grant AM Campbell MJ	1992	BMJ 304: 1030–2	1. Breast shells or 2. Hoffman's exercises or 3. Hoffman's exercises and breast shells versus 4. Neither breast shells or Hoffman's exercises	At least one inverted or non-protractile nipples Nulliparous Singleton pregnancy Intending to breastfeed No previous surgery to nipples Not already using any of the treatments Between 25–35 weeks of pregnancy	96	Sustained improvement in nipple anatomy Breastfeeding successfully at 6 weeks after delivery (This included women who were giving complementary or supplementary bottle feeds)	52% (25/48) of the women allocated to wearing breast shells showed sustained improvement compared to 60% (29/48) wearing no shells 54% (26/48) of those who were recommended exercises showed sustained improvement compared to 58% (28/48) who did not use exercises 29% (14/48) of those women who used shells were breastfeeding successfully at 6 weeks compared with 50% (24/48) of those women who did not use shells and were breastfeeding successfully at 6 weeks 40% (19/48) of those women who used exercises were breastfeeding successfully at 6 weeks compared with 40% (19/48) of those women who did not use exercises were breastfeeding successfully at 6 weeks

TABLE 13: Preparing for breastfeeding: treatment of inverted and non-protractile nipples in pregnancy

Method: Randomised controlled trial

Authors	Date	Where published	Intervention assessed	Entry criteria	Number of women studied	Outcomes measured	Results
The MAIN Trial Collaborative Group	1994	Midwifery 10(4): 200–214	1. Breast shells or 2. Hoffman's exercises or 3. Hoffman's exercises and breast shells versus 4. Neither breast shells or Hoffman's exercises	Women with at least one inverted or non-protractile nipple Singleton pregnancy Recruited between 25 completed – 35 completed weeks of pregnancy	463	Rate of breastfeeding as reported by postal questionnaire at 6 weeks postpartum	Allocated to Hoffman's exercises: 107/234 (46%) breastfeeding at 6 weeks Not allocated to Hoffman's exercises: 100/229 (44%) breastfeeding at 6 weeks Used breast shells: 103/230 (45%) breastfeeding at 6 weeks Did not use breast shells: 104/233 (45%) breastfeeding at 6 weeks

TABLE 14: The inverted nipple: to cut the ducts or not?

Method: Case studies

Authors	Date	Where published	Method	Entry criteria	Number of women studied	Outcomes measured	Results
Terrill PJ Stapleton MJ	1991	British Journal of Plastic Surgery 44: 372–377	1. Lactiferous ducts not divided (DND) six patients (9 nipples) 2. Lactiferous ducts completely divided (DCD) four patients (6 nipples)	Attended Plastic Surgery Unit, Victoria, Australia, in the 10 years between 1978–1987	26 women – only 5 were pregnant 44 nipples	Protrusion of their nipples Nipple sensitivity, response to cold and sexual arousal Ability to breastfeed	Nipple eversion was maintained in 59% of cases, with no difference in the rate of reinversion whether the ducts were divided (27%) or not (25%). Altered nipple sensation occured in 42% of cases, 33% in the DND group, 45% in DCD group of which 20% persisted (0% in DND group). Accordingly, there was permanent loss of nipple sensation in 20% of cases where the ducts were completely divided. Post operatively 5 women had children. Two did not breastfeed on advice of surgeon. Three attempted. Woman 1: DCD – able to breastfeed but with reduced lactation. Woman 2: DCD – breastfed with aid of nipple shields. Woman 3: DCD – unable to breastfeed.

TABLE 15: Treatment of inverted nipples using a disposable syringe

Method: Case studies

Authors	Date	Where published	Intervention assessed	Entry criteria	Number of women studied	Outcomes measured	Results
Kesaree N Banapurmath C R Banapurmath S Shamanur K	1993	J. Hum Lact 9(1): 27–9	Women used a modified 10ml plastic disposable syringe, cut and inverted so that the smooth end could be applied to the nipple, while manual withdrawal of the plunger would apply suction Suction was applied for 30 seconds or more before the baby attached to the breast The intervention also included: teaching effective positioning of the baby at the breast; discouragement of bottle-feeding; and the use of cup or spoon-feeding to give supplements	8 babies hospitalised with septicaemia, dehydration or broncho-pneumonia	8	Exclusive breastfeeding established	Six women proceeded to breastfeed successfully, doing so exclusively within 2–6 weeks A seventh baby, who was over 6 months old was both breastfed and received semi-solid foods The eighth mother "sought discharge after 8 days and was lost to follow-up"

TABLE 16: The 'Niplette': an instrument for the non-surgical correction of inverted nipples

Method: Case studies

Authors	Date	Where published	Intervention assessed	Entry criteria	Number of women studied	Outcomes measured	Results
McGeorge DD	1994	British Journal of Plastic Surgery 47: 46–49	Women using the 'Niplette'. The Niplette uses suction to stretch the lactiferous ducts gently. Nipple mould fitted over nipple areola complex. Air is withdrawn using a 8ml syringe	16 consecutive women referred to the regional Plastic Surgery Centre at Roehampton for consideration of surgical treatment of inverted nipples	16 +6 referred from antenatal clinic	Breastfeeding	"14 women who were pregnant, all breastfed without difficulty"

TABLE 17: Initiating breastfeeding: a world survey of the timing of postpartum breastfeeding

Method: Literature review

Authors	Date	Where published	Intervention assessed	Entry criteria	Number of women studied	Outcomes measured	Results
Morse JM Jehle C Gamble D	1990	Int J Nursing Studies 27(3): 303–313	A literature review was conducted All references to postnatal methods and beliefs of infant feeding were sorted according to the timing of the first feed	N/A	120 cultural groups	Length of time breastfeeding was withheld Substitute pre-lacteal foods Reasons for withholding colostrum	50 (41.7%) withheld the infant from the breast for >48 hours Water Water and glucose Infant formula 1. Dirty, poisonous, contaminated, bad or contained pus (16 groups) 2. Nothing, insufficient, or too hot (6 groups) 3. Would make the child ill, causing vomiting or diarrhoea (5 groups)

TABLE 18: An experiment to determine a basis for nursing decisions in regard to time of initiation of breastfeeding

Method: Non-randomised prospective comparison study

Authors	Date	Where published	Intervention assessed	Entry criteria	Number of women studied	Outcomes measured	Results
Eppink H	1969	Nursing Research 18(4): 292–99	Initiation of breastfeeding within 8 hours of delivery, compared with routine care (>24hr)	Healthy women intending to breastfeed, giving birth to a healthy baby weighing >6lb All babies received water by dropper before the first breastfeed, babies in the control group received 3 water feeds in the first 24hr	60 babies, assigned to experimental and control groups (30 in each) on alternate weekends 3 women allocated to experimental group elected to delay nursing, 12 babies failed to initiate breastfeeding when first offered (2 till >48hr old)	Latency to sucking at first breastfeed Weight loss of babies by post-partum day 3 Intake at a feed on day 3 Amount of formula taken (formula routinely given to both groups of babies at night) Difficulty with breathing in first 24hr	Significantly shorter latency to initiate breastfeeding in early contact group (p<0.01) (analysis by intention to treat, i.e. all 30 in each group) Weight loss 6.2oz in <8hr group versus 7.5oz in >24hr group (p<0.05) (analysis by completion of protocol, i.e. 24 in each group) Amount of breast-milk: 1.4oz in <8hr group, 1.1oz in >24hr group (not significant) Formula taken: 7.3oz in <8hr group, 11.0oz in >24hr group (p<0.05) Increased number of suctionings in first 24 hr in <8hr group (no significance level reported)

TABLE 19: Randomised trial: short-term effects of early suckling and touch of nipple on maternal behaviour

Method: Randomised trial

Authors	Date	Where published	Intervention assessed	Entry criteria	Number of women studied	Outcomes measured	Results
Widström A-M Wahlberg V Matthiesen A-S Encrom P Uvnäs-Moberg K Werner S Winberg J	1990	Early Human Development 21: 153–163	Early contact and suckling within 30 minutes of delivery versus Early contact and suckling according to hospital routine (approx. 8.8 hours after delivery)	Healthy Primiparous Uncomplicated vaginal delivery	57 primiparas 32 Experimental group 25 Control group	Infant's sucking ability	Experimental group: 6 (19%) of 32 infants sucked well at the first attempt Control group: 17 (73%) of infants sucked well at the first attempt
						Effects on maternal behaviour in the first week	Short breastfeeding observation on the 4th day. Significantly more in the experimental group (31/32) than in control (18/25) talked to their infants. Infants of those assigned to early suckling spent less time in the nursery
						Data on different aspects of breastfeeding and maternal mood	There was no significant difference regarding mothers' expectations and feelings about breastfeeding
						Prolactin and gastrin levels in maternal serum immediately before or after the second breastfeed on day 4	There was no statistical difference between the two groups

TABLE 20: Effect of early suckling on term neonates' core body temperature

Method: Randomised controlled trial

Authors	Date	Where published	Intervention assessed	Entry criteria	Number of women studied	Outcomes measured	Results
van den Bosch CA Bullough CHW	1990	Annals of Tropical Paediatrics 10: 347–353	Early suckling group – encouraged to breastfeed as soon as possible after birth Controls – normal management. The babies were placed in cots with a heated mattress and mothers breastfed when ready (usually after bathing and resting)	Babies born during the day at Kamazu Central Hospital, Malawi, Feb–Jun 1988 Excluded: Preterm <2000g Apgar <6 at 5 minutes. Babies with abnormalities. Babies who had had offensive liquor	160 81 early suckling 79 controls	Behaviour of the mothers towards the babies Clothing worn by the babies Rectal temperature after the thermometer had been in situ for 3 minutes, at 2 hours and 4 hours post delivery, and at 8am next day	No significant differences Differences had no significant effect on the babies' temperatures Significantly fewer of the early suckling group had temperatures below 36.5°C at 8am

TABLE 21: Duration of breastfeeding after early initiation and frequent feeding

Method: Randomised trial

Authors	Date	Where published	Intervention assessed	Entry criteria	Number of women studied	Outcomes measured	Results
Salariya EM Easton PM Cater JI	1978	Lancet ii: 1141–1143	4 groups, matched for age and social class. 2 groups fed within 10 minutes of birth, the other 2, 4–6 hours later	Primiparous Chose to breastfeed Term, healthy babies	111 at Ninewells Hospital, Dundee	When lactation started	At least 24 hours earlier in the 2-hour feeding groups
						Complementary feeds	Fewer given in the 2-hour groups
			One of each pair of groups then fed 2-hourly until lactation began, the other 4-hourly			Breastfeeding continuation: at 6 weeks at 12 weeks	Both slightly higher in the 2-hour groups
			Ward regimes for all the babies included complementary feeds and no night breastfeeds			If oral contraceptives being used	No effect on the discontinuation of breastfeeding
						Breastfeeding continuation at 18 months	Both early initiation and increased frequency extended the breastfeeding period. The wide range caused statistical problems; differences couldn't be expressed in terms of probability

TABLE 22: The initiation of lactation: the effect of early versus delayed contact for suckling on milk intake in the first week post-partum A study in Chiang Mai, Northern Thailand

Method: Randomised controlled trial

Authors	Date	Where published	Intervention assessed	Entry criteria	Number of women studied	Outcomes measured	Results
Woolridge M W Greasley V Silpisornkosol S	1985	Early Human Development 12: 269–78	Initiation of mother-infant contact and of the first breastfeed within 5hr of delivery versus routine care (>24hr to first contact)	Any healthy women delivering a healthy term infant (wt >2.5 kg) after an uncomplicated delivery	32 11 allocated to early contact group 7 to routine contact NB Heavy subject depletion forced departure from random-isation procedure	Milk transfer at a feed on days 2, 3, 4 & 5 post-partum	No significant differences were found in the onset of milk production over days 2–5 post-partum (ANOVA between groups – F=0.29, not signif.; across days – F=62.7, p<0.001; interaction between groups with time – F=0.02, not significant) *NB An observational study, conducted in parallel, highlighted the large proportion of time mothers spent in contact with or close proximity to their infants, amounting to 63% of the day and 95% of the night. Time spent breastfeeding increased from 10% during the day to 21% at night*

TABLE 23: Breast-feeding at one hour of age

Method: Prospective comparison study

Authors	Date	Where published	Intervention assessed	Entry criteria	Number of women studied	Outcomes measured	Results
Johnson N W	1976	The American Journal of Maternal Child Nursing 12–16	Initiation of breastfeeding within 1 hour of delivery (experimental), compared with 16hr or over (routine policy)	Not stated	12 6 in each group	Positive statements made by mothers about breastfeeding, equated with 'breastfeeding success' Prevalence of breastfeeding at 2 months of age	5/6 breastfed successfully in early breastfeeding (<1hr) group, compared with 1/6 successful in late breastfeeding (>16hr) group 5/6 still breastfeeding in <1hr group compared with 1/6 still breastfeeding in >16hr group

TABLE 24: The impact of a hospital and clinic-based breastfeeding promotion programme in a middle-class urban environment

Method: Non randomised prospective comparison study

Authors	Date	Where published	Intervention assessed	Entry criteria	Number of women studied	Outcomes measured	Results
Valdes V Perez A Labbock M Pugin E Zambrano I Catalan S	1993	Journal of Tropical Paediatrics 39: 142–151	Breastfeeding Promotion Programme (BPP) versus control group 4 steps: 1. Training of healthcare team in breastfeeding 2. Activities at prenatal clinic: -multimedia information -group discussions and individual teaching with nurse-trainer 3. Activities at hospital: -early breastfeeding -24hr rooming in -supplementary feeding reduced 4. Creation of open outpatient lactation clinic	1. Age 18–39 2. Parity up to 5 3. Healthy, no history of infertility 4. Couple in stable union 5. Work situation compatible with 6 months exclusive breastfeeding 6. Term, vaginal delivery, singleton birth, healthy, birthweight >2500 g 7. Written informed consent of the couple	313 controls 422 experimental group	Time from birth to first breastfed Frequency of supplementary feeds in hospital Supplementary feeds between going home and first clinic visit Using pacifiers (dummies) Reported problems with breastfeeding at first consultation Number of breastfeeds in 24 hours 1–6 months Duration of breastfeeds	Average 6.7 hours (controls) Average 2.8 hours (experimental group) 53% (controls) 19% (experimental group) 6.3% (controls) 1.6% (experimental group) 25.5% (controls) 15.1% (experimental group) 24% (controls) 31% (experimental group) Average 8–9 feeds (experimental group) shows a consistently higher average, (by 1–2 feeds/day) No difference between groups Average >160 mins/day in 1st month, about 120 mins/day in 6th month

TABLE 24: continued

Authors	Date	Where published	Intervention assessed	Entry criteria	Number of women studied	Outcomes measured	Results
			Subgroup received home visits			Exclusive breastfeeding at 6/12	31.6% controls 66.8% (experimental group)
						Exclusive breastfeeding and amenorrhoea	22% controls 56.2% (experimental group)
						Complete weaning at 6/12	23.3% controls 10.7% (experimental group)
						Solid supplements begun at 4 months	No difference between groups

TABLE 25: Effect of delivery room routines on success of first breast-feed

Method: Non-randomised comparison study

Authors	Date	Where published	Intervention assessed	Entry criteria	Number of women studied	Outcomes measured	Results
Righard L Alade M	1990	Lancet ii: 1105–1107	Uninterrupted contact between mother and baby for at least 1 hour versus Infant placed on the mother's abdomen immediately after birth but removed for weighing etc after 20 minutes	80 healthy mothers with uncomplicated pregnancies were enrolled consecutively Informed consent was obtained from 72 mothers	72 infants Contact group = 38 Separation group = 34	Sucking pattern and the effect of Pethidine	Contact group: All but 3 infants started making arm and leg movements after a mean 19.0 minutes in an attempt to reach the breast 24 of the 38 sucked correctly 4 sucked in a faulty manner. 10 did not suck at all (all 10 affected by Pethidine) Of 34 infants in separation group: 7 sucked correctly 11 sucked incorrectly 16 refused to suck Of the 26 infants who did not suck at all 25 were born to mothers sedated with Pethidine

TABLE 26: Impact and sustainability of a "baby-friendly" health education intervention at a district hospital in Bihar, India

Method: Non-randomised prospective study of intervention

Authors	Date	Where published	Intervention assessed	Entry criteria	Number of women studied	Outcomes measured	Results
Prasad B Costello AM de L	1995	BMJ 310: 621–623	10-day training programme for doctors, nurses and midwives, explaining benefits and feasibility of early breastfeeding, and the dangers of pre-lacteal feeds, with instructions on teaching this to mothers 172 mothers were interviewed pre-intervention 195 mothers were interviewed immediately post-intervention 101 mothers were interviewed six months later	SVD of healthy singleton or twins at Sadar district hospital	468 Control: 172 pre-intervention Experiment 1: 195 immediately post-intervention Experiment 2: 101 6 months later	Age of infant when breastfeeding started Number of mothers using pre-lacteal feeds Colostrum feeding	Breastfeeding started earlier and fewer pre-lacteal feeds were used immediately post-intervention Control group: 165/172 (96%) were using pre-lacteal feeds Experiment 1 group: 84/195 (43%) were using pre-lacteal feeds Experiment 2 group: 78/101 (77%) were using pre-lacteal feeds 6 months later, the improvement in outcomes was not sustained and many mothers were not receiving teaching Staff updates were recommended

TABLE 27: Study of factors promoting and inhibiting lactation

Method: Non randomised, prospective, controlled studies

Authors	Date	Where published	Intervention assessed	Entry criteria	Number of women studied	Outcomes measured	Results
de Chateau P Holmberg H Jakobsson K Winberg J	1977	Develop Med Child Neurol 19: 575–584	Studies made between 1972–1975	Healthy, full-term newborn infants			
			1. Control infants weighed before and after suckling, supplementary feeding during the 1st week versus not weighing, not giving supplementary feeds	Born Feb–Mar 1972 Born Apr–Jun 1972 Born May 1973	Part I: 390 infants 119 in control group 203 in group I 68 in group II	Part I: Weight development Duration of breastfeeding	No significant difference between groups No significant difference in duration control versus group I, median 42 and 47 days. Controls five times more likely to stop breastfeeding in 1st week. Median duration for group II longer than controls by 95 days (p<0.0005)
			2. Increased information and support to mothers and fathers, with extended postnatal support. Test group A had routine + additional information; test group B also had prolonged postnatal support	Born in 1974 to primiparous mothers	Part II: 66 infants 23 in control group 23 in test group A 20 in test group B	Part II: Duration of breastfeeding and early failure Effect of informing fathers	No significant difference in duration, but if they had additional information 'early failure' was reduced from 28% to 6% If fathers were informed median number of days was 135. If fathers were not informed, median number of days was 75
			3. Immediate postpartum skin-to-skin contact and sucking between mother and infant versus short glimpse of infant and then taken away (routine care)	Born 1974/75 Healthy full-term infants of primiparas	Part III: 42 infants 20 in control received routine care 22 in study group	Part III: Duration of breastfeeding Behavioural and psychological effects	Median of 108 days in control group, 175 days in study group. Boys fed longer in both groups Mothers in the study group gave night feed for a median of 42 days. In control groups the median was 24 days

TABLE 28: Gastric suction in healthy newborn infants

Method: Prospective randomised study

Authors	Date	Where published	Intervention assessed	Entry criteria	Number of women studied	Outcomes measured	Results
Widström A-M Ransjö-Arvidson A-B Christensson K Matthiesen A-S Winberg J Uvnäs-Moberg K	1987	Acta Paediatr Scand 76: 566–572	Experimental group: gastric suction for 5–6 minutes after birth Control group: no gastric suction Randomly allocated No mucus extraction from airways	Healthy Term Birthweight 3000–4000g	21 11 cases 10 controls	*Immediate:* -Blood pressure -Heart rate -Defensive movements -Retching *3–4 hours:* -Spont. sucking/rooting movements -State of sleep and wakefulness *1–4 days:* -Feeding/vomiting -Weight	Significant rise in experimental group No difference Made by 9/11 in experimental group More by babies in experimental group Disrupted in experimental group No difference No difference No difference Concludes: The physiological side-effects produced by gastric suction are minor, but it seemed to be unpleasant for the child and no clear advantages are gained by the procedure

TABLE 29: Sore nipples: causes and prevention

Method: Prospective study

Authors	Date	Where published	Intervention assessed	Entry criteria	Number of women studied	Outcomes measured	Results
Gunther M	1945	Lancet ii: 590–593	Prospective study Observational investigation of pressure changes within the babies' mouths during sucking Whether oral ascorbic acid reduces incidence of sore nipples Measurements made of infant oral suction pressure	Breastfeeding in first 5 days Infant weighing >6lb	400 preliminary observation 114 detailed study	Incidence of sore nipples Types of lesion Soreness and capillary resistance	64% of 114 women experienced sore nipples Two common types were identified; erosive (petechial) and ulcerative (fissure) No significant correlation found between the incidence of soreness and capillary resistance, Vitamin C supplement and parity The nipple pain varied with baby's weight, however, with sore nipples being more common with larger babies 'than would be expected by chance'

TABLE 30: Sucking technique and its effect on success of breastfeeding

Method: Randomised controlled trial

Authors	Date	Where published	Intervention assessed	Entry criteria	Number of women studied	Outcomes measured	Results
Righard L Alade M	1992	Birth 19(4): 185–189	Breastfeeding technique was observed at discharge (4–6 days) by the same observer. Natural Control Group, where mother/infant pairs were identified as having a correct sucking technique were consecutively selected. When an incorrect or nipple sucking technique was identified, the mother/infant pair were randomly assigned to one of two groups: 1. Nipple sucking (NS) group – sucking technique not corrected 2. Corrected group	Breastfeeding. Delivered at the University Hospitals of Malmö and Lund. Women with a correct breastfeeding technique were consecutively selected as controls	82 NS group = 25 Corrected = 29 Controls = 28	Exclusive and partial breastfeeding during: Month 1 Month 2 Month 3 Month 4 Incidence of breastfeeding problems Milk insufficiency reported Use of pacifier	NS Group 'Correct*' 64% 96% p<0.001 48% 84% p<0.01 44% 79% p<0.01 40% 74% p<0.01 *'Correct' sucking controls and 'corrected' group combined (n=28+29=57), data for these two groups not reported separately 88% 53% p<0.001 Significantly more in NS group (p<0.05) Breastfeeding problems were more commonly reported by mothers using a pacifier >2hrs/day Pacifiers were used by 40% of the mothers still breastfeeding at 4 months, but by 90% of those who had already stopped

TABLE 31: Positive effects of an antenatal group teaching session on postnatal nipple pain, nipple trauma and breast feeding rates

Method: Randomised trial (pilot study)

Authors	Date	Where published	Intervention assessed	Entry criteria	Number of women studied	Outcomes measured	Results
Duffy E P Percival P Kershaw E	1997	Midwifery 13: 189–96	An antenatal teaching session on positioning and attachment	Pregnant women (36 weeks gestation) intending to breastfeed	75 women 37 allocated to experimental group and 38 to control group	Assessment of positioning and attachment using an observational tool (LATCH – scales from 0–10)	Higher LATCH score for experimental group (mean score across first 4 post-natal days = 8.8) than for control group (mean = 6.0), indicating better positioning and attachment (ANOVA p<0.001*)
						Nipple pain using a visual analogue scale (VAS – scales from 0–10)	Lower VAS score for experimental group (mean score across first 4 postnatal days = 0.9) than for control group (mean = 5.9) indicating significantly less nipple pain (ANOVA p<0.001)
						Nipple trauma measured using a nipple trauma index (NTI – scales from 0–34, higher values mean less trauma)	Higher NTI measures in experimental group (mean score across first 4 postnatal days = 33.2) than for control group (mean = 23.6) indicating significantly less nipple trauma experienced (ANOVA p<0.001*)
						Breastfeeding outcome at 6 weeks	92% of experimental group fully breastfeeding at 6 weeks compared with 29% of control group (p<0.001) * indicates there is also a significant Group by Day interaction

TABLE 32: A double-blind controlled trial of chlorhexidine in aerosol spray for the prevention of sore nipples

Method: A double-blind trial using coded drugs

Authors	Date	Where published	Intervention assessed	Entry criteria	Number of women studied	Outcomes measured	Results
Slaven S Craft I Harvey DR	1988	Unpublished	Chlorhexidine spray versus a placebo for the prevention of sore nipples	Breastfeeding women	723	Incidence of sore nipples	Experimental group: 126/370 (34%) women developed sore nipples Control group: 116/346 (33%) women developed sore nipples
						Cracked nipples	Experimental group: 58/370 (15%) women developed cracked nipples Control group: 59/346 (17%) women developed cracked nipples
						Breast engorgement	Experimental group: 76/370 (20%) women developed engorged breasts Control group: 62/346 (17%) women developed engorged breasts

TABLE 33: Two aerosol sprays in nipple trauma

Method: A randomised trial using unmarked spray cans

Authors	Date	Where published	Intervention assessed	Entry criteria	Number of women studied	Outcomes measured	Results
Herd B Feeney JG	1986	Practitioner 230: 31–38	Chlorhexidine spray versus placebo for the prevention of nipple discomfort and trauma	Women who wished to breastfeed; having had a normal delivery with both the mother and infant in good health. Women were excluded if they had previously had an adverse reaction to the test medications; taking drugs which could be expressed in breastmilk; or who were unlikely to persevere with breastfeeding	200	Duration of breastfeeding	Experimental group: 4/100 women stopped breastfeeding in the first 2 weeks following delivery Control group: 7/100 women stopped breastfeeding in the first 2 weeks Experimental group: 18/100 women stopped breastfeeding in the first 4 weeks following delivery Control group: 31/100 women stopped breastfeeding in the first 4 weeks
						Nipple trauma	Experimental group: 7/100 women experienced severe nipple trauma 1 week following delivery 24/100 women experienced mild trauma Control group: 4/100 women experienced severe nipple trauma 1 week following delivery 38/100 women experienced mild trauma
						Oral thrush in the infant	Experimental group: 7/100 babies developed oral thrush Control group: 8/100 babies developed oral thrush

TABLE 34: A study in nipple care

Method: Non-randomised prospective comparison study

Authors	Date	Where published	Intervention assessed	Entry criteria	Number of women studied	Outcomes measured	Results
Rickitt C	1986	Midwives Chronicle and Nursing Notes 131–132	Nipple care comparison between Rotersept spray and expressed breast milk	Breastfeeding women on two different wards, treatment allocated by ward	98	Numbers of mothers on 6th day who experienced cracked nipples	No significant difference was found in the incidence of sore nipples on the two wards by which treatment was allocated

TABLE 35: The effectiveness of topical agents in reducing nipple soreness of breastfeeding mothers

Method: Non-randomised prospective comparison study

Authors	Date	Where published	Intervention assessed	Entry criteria	Number of women studied	Outcomes measured	Results
Riordan J	1985	J Hum Lact 1(3): 36–41	1. Right or left breast, decided by flip of a coin: treat sore nipples with lanolin or tea bags 2. Control breast: treat with nothing	Primagravida Over 18 years Singleton Normal postpartum	20	Pain in the morning and the evening of the first 6 days postpartum	No significant difference. Topical treatments of nipples of lactating women are not effective in alleviating nipple soreness

TABLE 36: Comfort measures in breastfeeding, primiparous women

Method: Prospectively randomised trial

Authors	Date	Where published	Intervention assessed	Entry criteria	Number of women studied	Outcomes measured	Results
Buchko BL Pugh LC Bishop BA Cochran JF Smith LR Lerew DJ	1993	JOGNN 23(1): 46–52	All mothers in the trial received instruction regarding breastfeeding. In addition they were assigned to one of the following treatments 1. Warm moist tea-bag compress 2. Warm water compress 3. Expressed breast milk massaged into nipple and areola and air dried 4. Instruction only Mothers completed questionnaire daily x7 days	Breastfeeding primiparous women 18 years or older English speaking Telephone at home Low risk pregnancy Vaginal delivery of a singleton Term healthy infant	94	Effect of treatment on postpartum nipple soreness	Warm water was the most effective method of alleviating the pain Nipple pain was highest on postpartum days 3 and 4 No women in the control (Instruction only group) switched to formula feeding There was no significant difference between the other groups

TABLE 37: A comparison of topical agents to relieve nipple pain and enhance breastfeeding

Method: Randomised comparison study

Authors	Date	Where published	Intervention assessed	Entry criteria	Number of women studied	Outcomes measured	Results
Pugh L C Buchko B L Bishop B A Cochran J F Smith L R Lerew D J	1996	Birth 23(2): 88–93	All women received a formal breastfeeding educational plan Women were then randomly allocated to a treatment group 1. USP – modified lanolin 2. Warm water compresses 3. Expressed breastmilk with air drying 4. Breastfeeding educational programme only	Breastfeeding women over 18 years Primipara Low risk pregnancy, labour and delivery Term healthy infant Telephone in home and English speaking	177 Group 1: 45 Group 2: 44 Group 3: 44 Group 4: 44	1. Nipple soreness on days 4, 7 and 14 2. Breastfeeding discontinuation at 6 weeks	No significant differences in pain intensity, pain affect or duration of breastfeeding was shown between groups Logistic regression indicated that older mothers and those who were exclusively breastfeeding at 14 days, were most likely to be breastfeeding at 6 weeks

TABLE 38: Does application of tea bags to sore nipples while breastfeeding provide effective relief?

Method: A single-blind randomised controlled trial

Authors	Date	Where published	Intervention assessed	Entry criteria	Number of women studied	Outcomes measured	Results
Lavergne N A	1997	JOGNN 26(1): 53–58	Women were randomly assigned two out of the three treatments: 1. Tea bag compress 2. Water compress 3. No compress The two treatments were further randomly assigned to either the right or left nipple	Breastfeeding primiparous women who had had a vaginal delivery at term.	65 Attrition rate 44% 21: bags versus compresses 22: nothing versus compresses 22: bags versus nothing	Nipple pain, self-rated on a 6-point scale (0=no pain, 1–5= increasing intensity of pain) Median of pain rating after at least 4 feeds per day	Tea bags and warm water compresses were equally effective at reducing nipple pain [Graphical portrayal of the results suggests that the tea bag and nothing groups showed a reduction in nipple pain from day 2 to day 5, while the warm water compress group still showed elevated pain on day 5 (the results reported are discrepant with figure 1, suggesting that it may be incorrect).]

TABLE 39: Self-demand feeding in a maternity unit

Method: Non-randomised prospective comparison study

Authors	Date	Where published	Intervention assessed	Entry criteria	Number of women studied	Outcomes measured	Results
Illingworth RS Stone DGH Jowett GH Scott JF	1952	Lancet i: 683–87	A 'self demand' schedule versus a rigid 4-hourly schedule	Breastfeeding women and their infants Preterm infants and infants with cerebral irritation were excluded	137	Infant weight gain (regained birth weight by 9th day)	56/114 (49.1%) in the demand fed group had regained their birth weight 35/97 (36.1%) in the rigid feeding group had regained their birth weight
						Breast discomfort:	
						Sore nipples	29/106 (27.4%) of those in rigid group complained of sore nipples compared with 16/124 (12.9%) of women in the demand group
						Breast engorgement	36/106 (34%) of those in rigid group complained of engorgement compared with 21/124 (16.9%) of those women in the demand group
						Sore nipples and engorgement	Incidence of both sore nipples and engorgement was 3.6 times more likely in the rigid group than in the demand fed group (5.7% versus 1.6%)
						Number of feeds in 24 hours in the 'self-demand' group	5th postpartum day 36/124 (28.6%) infants demanded >7 feeds per day
							5th postpartum day 12/124 (9.5%) infants demanded >9 feeds per day
							7th postpartum day 20/124 (15.5%) of infants demanded >8 feeds per day

TABLE 40: Does the duration and frequency of early breastfeeding effect nipple pain?

Method: Non-randomised prospective study

Authors	Date	Where published	Intervention assessed	Entry criteria	Number of women studied	Outcomes measured	Results
de Carvalho M Robertson S Klaus MH	1984	Birth 11(2): 81–84	To assess the effect of frequency and duration of breastfeeding on the development of sore nipples Comparison: Control group fed 3–4 hourly timed feeds Experimental group fed on demand, in days 1–10 postpartum	Normal delivery at term	32	Nipple soreness in two comparison groups Feed frequency	No significant difference in nipple soreness in either group, although nipple pain decreased in both groups from days 1–5 to days 6–10 Mothers in experimental group fed more frequently (10 versus 7.4 feeds per 24 hr, p<0.0001) *NB 73% of women in study experienced slight to moderate discomfort, which peaked on the third day post-partum and declined rapidly thereafter. As nipple soreness decreased over the time when feed frequency increased, the authors concluded that "frequent feedings in early lactation do not increase the incidence of nipple discomfort."*

TABLE 41: Effect of frequent breastfeeding on early milk production and infant weight gain

Method: Non-randomised prospective comparison study

Authors	Date	Where published	Intervention assessed	Entry criteria	Number of women studied	Outcomes measured	Results
de Carvalho M Robertson S Friedman A Klaus M	1983	Pediatrics 72(3): 307–311	Experimental group: encouraged to nurse frequently (n=20) Control group: nursed 3–4 hourly (n=24)	Uncomplicated delivery at Mount Sinai Medical Centre, Cleveland Intended to breastfeed Delivered July/August (controls) Delivered Sept/Oct (experimental group) Consented	47 women enrolled Sample reduced to 24 women by day 15 (reasons for drop-out given) Sample further reduced to 16 women by day 35 Babies in experimental group were 478g heavier at birth on average than control infants	Length and time of each feed 1–14 days Milk intake per feed and weight gain from birth on: Day 15 Day 35	The experimental group nursed significantly more frequently, 9.9±1.9 feeds/24hr, compared with 8.3±1.4 in the control group (p<0.0001), although the mean duration of breastfeeding/24h was similar (134 versus 138 min/24h) More feeds were also given on day 35 (9.8±2.4 versus 6.8±1.2, p>0.01) The experimental group babies took significantly more milk (725±171g versus 502±185g, p<0.001) and gained significantly more weight (561±286g versus 347±331g, p<0.02) There were no significant differences in either milk intake (841±285 versus 681±179g) or weight gain (1,350±418 versus 1,246±356g) by 35th day

TABLE 42: Breastfeeding of term infants

Method: Randomised trial

Authors	Date	Where published	Intervention assessed	Entry criteria	Number of women studied	Outcomes measured	Results
Gale R Dollberg S Branski D Stevenson DK Seidman DS	1989	Clinical Pediatrics 28(10): 458–460	3-hourly feeding schedule versus 4-hourly feeding schedule The 2am feed in both groups was a formula feed given by the nursing staff	Breastfeeding Term, singleton infants with birth weights between 2500–2990 g	152 90 in 4-hourly group 62 in 3-hourly group	Infant weight loss on: Day 1 Day 2 Mean serum bilirubin levels	Mean weight loss on day 1 3-hourly group = 91.8±64.2 grams Mean weight loss on day 1 4-hourly group = 102.7±68.9 grams Mean weight loss on day 2 3-hourly group = 41.0±62.8 grams Mean weight loss on day 2 4-hourly group = 29.4±52.5 grams 138±47 mg/dl in 3-hourly group 133±47 mg/dl in 4-hourly group

TABLE 43: How long should a breastfeed last?

Method: Non-randomised prospective study

Authors	Date	Where published	Intervention assessed	Entry criteria	Number of women studied	Outcomes measured	Results
Howie PJ Houston MJ Cook A Smart L McArdle T McNeilly AS	1981	Early Human Development 5: 71–77	Babies weighed before feed and at 5-minute intervals during feed for two consecutive feeds between days 5–7 Mothers were asked to give, either: One feed for 10 minutes from each breast (10x10) or One feed for 5 minutes from each breast x2 (5x5x5)	Babies born in Simpson Memorial Maternity Pavilion, Edinburgh Birthweight >2800g Mothers breastfeeding on demand	50	Milk intakes Prolactin studies (10 women) Inter/intra patient variation Duration of feeds	The mean final milk intake did not differ significantly in either group In both regimes, 70% from the first breast and 80% of the milk from the second was taken during the first 5 minutes The sucking induced prolactin responses did not differ significantly between the regimes Wide variation Duration of suckling in 100 breastfeeding episodes showed wide variation between individuals and a high incidence of non nutritive suckling towards the end of a feed 'It is recommended that mothers should be told of the highly individual nature of breastfeeding and should be encouraged to time their feeds according to the responses of their own infants'

TABLE 44: Individual patterns of milk intake during breastfeeding

Method: Prospective study

Authors	Date	Where published	Intervention assessed	Entry criteria	Number of women studied	Outcomes measured	Results
Woolridge MW Baum JD Drewett RF	1982	Early Human Development 7:265–272 *also Perinatal Nutrition, chapter 19. Academic Press Inc, 1988*	Babies weighed: - before feed, - 4 minutes into a feed (1 or both breasts) - at the end of the feed (1 or both breasts)	Not referred to	20 babies 6 days old 2 babies (cousins) cross fed by their mothers/ aunts (sisters)	Milk intake at points specified, and therefore rate of transfer	Very varied both in feed length and rate of milk transfer, therefore 'rules' about the length of a breastfeed can only be guidelines not principles Suggests the rate of milk transfer for a mother-infant pair is determined both by the rate of milk release by the mother and the rate of milk demand by the baby

TABLE 45: Supplementary feeding and jaundice in newborns

Method: Randomised trial

Authors	Date	Where published	Intervention assessed	Entry criteria	Number of women studied	Outcomes measured	Results
Nicoll A Ginsberg R Tripp JH	1982	Acta Paediatr Scand 71: 759–761	1. Water supplementation or 2. Dextrose supplementation versus 3. No supplementation	Mothers intending to breastfeed term infants 5 day minimum hospital stay	49 enrolled, 2 later excluded Group 1: n=14 Group 2: n=17 Group 3: n=16	Supplements (ml/kg/day) taken (mean±SE)	Group 1 Group 2 Group 3 16.2±2.0 38.6±4.4 nil Differences in supplementation between groups was significant (p<0.001)
						Mean infant weight loss (%±SE) on: Day 3	Group 1 Group 2 Group 3 5.9±0.4 4.1±0.4 6.0±0.5 Dextrose group lost significantly less weight (significance level not reported)
						Day 5	Group 1 Group 2 Group 3 4.2±0.6 4.0±0.5 4.3±0.6 Differences not significant
						Serum bilirubin levels (SBR in μmol/l) on post-partum day 6 (mean±SE)	Group 1 Group 2 Group 3 93.5±13.8 80.8±8.8 67.7±6.7 Differences not significant
						Breast milk intake at a feed on day 6	Differences between groups not significant

TABLE 46: Hyperbilirubinaemia in breast-fed newborn: A controlled trial of four interventions

Method: Randomised trial

Authors	Date	Where published	Intervention assessed	Entry criteria	Number of women studied	Outcomes measured	Results
Martinez JC Maisels JM Otheguy L Garcia H Savorani M Mogni B Martinez JC (jnr)	1993	Pediatrics 91(2): 470–473	Group 1: Breastfeeding and observe Group 2: Discontinue breastfeeding, give formula Group 3: Discontinue breastfeeding, give formula and phototherapy Group 4: Continue breastfeeding, give phototherapy	Healthy term infants Mothers having had an uncomplicated pregnancy Serum bilirubin >291 μmol/L	125 Group 1=25 Group 2=26 Group 3=38 Group 4=36	Mean serum bilirubin not rising above 342 μmol/L	No significant difference between the groups There was no significant difference in the levels of serum bilirubin in the groups that continued breastfeeding to the groups that discontinued feeding

TABLE 47: Effects of water supplementation on physiological jaundice in breastfed babies

Method: Non-randomised, prospective, comparison study

Authors	Date	Where published	Intervention assessed	Entry criteria	Number of women studied	Outcomes measured	Results
de Carvalho M Hall M Harvey D	1981	Arch Dis Child 56: 568–569	Water supplementation given after each breastfeed versus no supplementation given	UK: Infants considered to have physiological jaundice, defined as a serum bilirubin at 200 μmol/l; term healthy infants with birthweights greater than 2.5kg	175	Serum bilirubin levels (SBR)	Experimental group n=120 mean SBR = 260 μmol/l Control group n=55 mean SBR = 263.50 μmol/l
						Number of infants requiring phototherapy	Experimental group n=120 11 infants required phototherapy Control group n=55 8 infants required phototherapy

TABLE 48: The relationship of breastfeeding to third day bilirubin levels

Method: Non-randomised prospective study

Authors	Date	Where published	Intervention assessed	Entry criteria	Number of women studied	Outcomes measured	Results
Johnson CA Lieberman B Hassanein RE	1985	Journal of Family Practice 20(2): 147–152	Serum bilirubin measured on day 3 Weight measured on day 3 Phototherapy if Serum bilirubin <15 mg/dl or above	Inclusion: Full term healthy babies born at study hospital between Oct–Nov 1980 and Jan–Feb 1981 Birth weight >2250g Cord blood Coomb's negative Exclusion: Cephalohaem-atoma, sepsis, baby needing special care/medication Babies of diabetic mothers	281 babies	Feeding method: breast, formula, mixed Serum bilirubin on 3rd day (and any other Serum bilirubin taken) Weight on the 3rd day	Lowest for formula and highest for breast p<0.01 Mean weight loss 180g for breastfed babies 100g for formula fed Weight loss was a significant predictor of higher Serum bilirubin on day 3 All breastfeeding mothers were given the option of offering sterile water to the infant after nursing. The amount of sterile water ingested bore no statistically significant relationship to the 3rd day bilirubin level. Breastfed infants receiving more than 60cc of formula or more than one formula feeding during the hospital stay were placed in the mixed-fed category

TABLE 49: Unsupplemented breastfeeding in the maternity ward

Method: Pre- & post-intervention study

Authors	Date	Where published	Intervention assessed	Entry criteria	Number of women studied	Outcomes measured	Results	
Nylander G Lindemann R Helsing E Bendvold E	1991	Acta Obstet Gynecol Scand 70: 205–9	Abandoning routine supplementation with sucrose solution and formula (replaced by water and/or pasteurised expressed breast milk (past.EBM)), and encouraging both early initiation and frequent breastfeeding	407 consecutive deliveries admitted to a single maternity ward, in a Norwegian hospital 204 mother-infant pairs before intervention, 203 after	Mothers with healthy term newborns	Process outcomes on second day:	Before mean (range)	After
						Breastfeeds/24hr	4.3 (1–6)	6.4 (3–10)
						Supplementary feeds/24hr	4.8 (4–8)	1.1 (0–3)
						Volume of breast milk consumed	47 ml (0–180)	132 ml (0–210)
						Volume of supplementary fluid consumed	188 ml (20–390)	23 ml (0–140)
							Before	After
						Non-milk supplementation percent received	100% sucrose	2% 'pure water'
						Amount taken in first 3 days	565 ml (165–1250)	68 ml (5–375)
							Before	After
						Milk supplementation percent received	81% formula	12% past. EBM
						Total amount taken during stay on maternity ward	170 ml (16–>1000)	75 ml (15–370)

TABLE 49: *continued*

Authors	Date	Where published	Intervention assessed	Entry criteria	Number of women studied	Outcomes measured	Results
						Outcomes of intervention:	
						% exclusive breastfeeding at:	Before After
						1.5 months	76% 93% p<0.001
						3 months	57% 75% p<0.001
						6 months	12% 22% p<0.01
						9 months	5% 7% n.s.
						% partial breastfeeding at:	Before After
						1.5 months	94% 96% n.s.
						3 months	88% 97% p<0.001
						6 months	66% 87% p<0.001
						9 months	47% 62% p<0.01
							Before After
						Duration of exclusive breastfeeding in months	3.5 (±2.1) 4.5 (±1.8) p<0.001
						Total duration of breastfeeding	6.9 (±3.3) 8.0 (±2.4) p<0.01

TABLE 50: Single daily bottle use in early weeks postpartum and breastfeeding

Method: Prospective randomised trial

Authors	Date	Where published	Intervention assessed	Entry criteria	Number of women studied	Outcomes measured	Results
Cronenwett L Stukel T Kearny M Barrett J Covington C del Monte K Reinhardt R Rippe L	1992	Pediatrics 90(5): 760–766	Single daily bottle given in weeks 2–6 postpartum (at least 5 days per week) ('planned bottle group') versus full breastfeeding, with mothers avoiding using bottles ('total breastfeeding group')	Women committed to breastfeeding for at least 6 weeks White married women Primiparous Attended childbirth classes	121 63 in the 'planned bottle group' 58 in the 'total breastfeeding group'	Prevalence of breastfeeding at 12 weeks 6 months	52/63 (83%) were still breastfeeding in the 'planned bottle group' compared with 54/58 (93%) of the total breastfeeding group' 37/63 (59%) were still breastfeeding in the 'planned bottle group' compared with 40/58 (68%) of the 'total breastfeeding group' Neither difference was significant

TABLE 51: The effect of feeding glucose water to breastfeeding newborns on weight, body temperature blood glucose and breastfeeding duration

Method: Randomised trial

Authors	Date	Where published	Intervention assessed	Entry criteria	Number of women studied	Outcomes measured	Results
Martin-Calama J Buñuel J Valero T Labay M Lasarte J J Valle F & de Miguel C	1997	J Hum Lact 13(3): 209–213	Supplementing breastfed newborns with glucose water by bottle	All women intending to breastfeed their full-term newborn, who had been delivered vaginally; and who had no congenital abnormality and no detectable risk factors for an abnormal blood glucose level Mothers excluded: Those planning to stop breastfeeding before 3 months post-partum; those receiving medication while in hospital; and those who did not follow "recommended baby friendly care steps" of hospital	180 GW: Glucose water group, n=83 NGW: No glucose water group, n=87 Outcomes measured in hospital, with follow-up after discharge at 5 months of age	Weight loss at 6, 12, 24, 48 and 72 hr of age Body temperature Serum glucose at 6, 12, 24, 48 and 72 hr of age Percentage of mothers who had introduced formula by age of baby	hrs GW NGW p 6 39.4 46.4 <0.05 12 74.9 86.4 <0.05 24 127.2 140.6 <0.05 48 165.3 197.8 <0.01 72 144.9 141.9 NS Mean max. temperature 37.3°C 37.4°C <0.05 Mean min. temperature 36.5°C 36.6°C <0.05 hrs GW NGW 6 3.68 3.39 <0.05 12 3.73 3.26 <0.001 24 3.73 3.39 <0.05 48 3.78 3.54 <0.01 Significantly more episodes of 'hypoglycaemia' detected at 12 hr of age (p<0.05) wks GW NGW 4 34% 19% <0.05 8 52% 38% NS 12 61% 44% NS 16 69% 60% NS 20 75% 70% NS

TABLE 52: The effect of extra fluid intake by breastfed babies in hospital on the duration of breastfeeding. Comparison of 3 regimes on different wards.

Method: Non-randomised prospective study

Authors	Date	Where published	Intervention assessed	Entry criteria	Number of women studied	Outcomes measured	Results
Houston MJ Howie PW McNeilly AS	1984	Journal of Reproductive and Infant Psychology 1: 42–48	Ward A: Demand feeding and clear fluids when mother felt baby would not settle Ward B: Demand feeding and clear or milk feeds after every breastfeed for the first 6 days Ward C: Demand feeding and clear or milk fluids, but not routinely as in Ward B	Breastfeeding mothers admitted to wards A, B, or C in the 3-week study period Babies needing special care and multiple births, excluded	70 A = 26 B = 26 C = 27	Demographic details from notes (including social class) Number of feeds Volume of extra fluids Duration of breastfeeding Jaundice	Women in social class I and II fed longer Significantly more on ward A on day 1 There were no significant differences thereafter Significantly less in ward A. Ward B gave significantly more on day 2, otherwise B and C similar No ward difference for women in social class I and II In classes III, IV and V more ward C women were feeding at 14 weeks No differences

TABLE 53: Effect of formula supplementation in the hospital on the duration of breast-feeding

Method: Non-randomised prospective comparison study

Authors	Date	Where published	Intervention assessed	Entry criteria	Number of women studied	Outcomes measured	Results
Gray-Donald K Kramer MS Munday S Leduc DG	1985	Pediatrics 75: 514–518	Restricted supplementation versus traditional supplementation practice Mothers in the restricted supplementation group were routinely woken to feed their babies at 2AM, the babies were given no formula supplements, unless requested by the mother. The use of glucose feeds was not restricted Mothers in the traditional routine supplementation group, gave a formula feed at 2AM. If infants had difficulty sucking or seemed hungry after a feed, formula was also offered	Full term, healthy babies Weighing more than 2500 kg	781	Proportion of infants who did not receive any supplements in hospital Infant weight loss in hospital Duration of breast feeding	Experiment group = 63.1% of infants in the restricted nursery did not receive any supplements Control group = 15% of infants in the traditional nursery did not receive any supplements Experiment group infants lost mean of 6% of their birth weight Control group infants lost mean 5.1% of their birth weight At 4 weeks Experiment group = 70.7% still breastfeeding Control group = 67.8% still breastfeeding At 9 weeks Experiment group = 54.7% still breastfeeding Control group = 54.1% still breastfeeding Babies who were still breastfeeding at 4 weeks and 9 weeks were more unlikely to have been unsupplemented 19.4% versus 4.4% at 4 weeks 20.9% versus 7.9% at 9 weeks

TABLE 54: Supplementary feeding in the maternity ward shortens the duration of breastfeeding

Method: Survey

Authors	Date	Where published	Intervention assessed	Entry criteria	Number of women studied	Outcomes measured	Results
Blomquist HK Jonsbo F Serenius F Persson LA	1994	Acta Paediatrica 83: 1122–6	A survey of feeding routines in a maternity unit, Umea, Sweden Feeding patterns of newborns were examined at 1,2,3 and 4 months	Born at University Hospital, Umea, Sweden, Feb–Apr 1990 Cared for mainly or wholly on the maternity ward	521 newborns	Risk of not being breastfed at 3 months in relation to feeding patterns in early neonatal period	At 3 months: 65% wholly breastfed 15% partially breastfed 20% not breastfed Not being breastfed at 3 months associated with maternal age (<25), maternal smoking, initial weight loss and early supplements Ward routines have changed since the study, with regard to supplements, rooming in, and use of breast pump and oxytocin spray

TABLE 55: UNICEF/WHO baby-friendly hospital initiative: does the use of bottles and pacifiers in the neonatal nursery prevent successful breastfeeding?

Method: Randomised controlled trial

Authors	Date	Where published	Intervention assessed	Entry criteria	Number of women studied	Outcomes measured	Results
Schubiger G Schwarz U Tönz O	1997	European Journal of Pediatrics 156: 874–7	Restricting fluid supplements and avoidance of bottles during first 5 days post-partum versus conventional hospital policy. Supplements, if medically indicated, given by cup/spoon in intervention group (teats and pacifiers forbidden) Standard care: supplements conventionally offered by bottle after breastfeeds (pacifiers also permitted)	Women, from 10 Swiss hospitals, intending to breastfeed for at least 3 months Healthy term newborns For eligibility, all hospitals to have established breastfeeding programmes, including at least 3 of WHO/UNICEF "Ten Steps"	602 women Group 1: UNICEF protocol n=294, 180 completed protocol, 114 (39%) violated protocol Group 2: Standard care n=308, 291 completed protocol, 17 (5.5%) violated protocol	Extra fluids given in first 5 days Prevalence of breastfeeding at: 2 months 4 months: 6 months:	Group 1: 165/180 (91.7%) infants received supplements of dextrin-maltose or formula Group 2: 281/289 (97.2%) infants received supplements of dextrin-maltose or formula Group 1 = 88.0% Group 2 = 87.7% not significant Group 1 = 75.4% Group 2 = 70.5% not significant Group 1 = 57.0% Group 2 = 55.3% not significant No differences in mean neonatal weight loss (−5.8% versus −5.5%), or the incidence of fever (0.6% versus 1.0%), phototherapy (2.2% versus 3.1%), or symptomatic hypoglycaemia (nil % in both groups)

TABLE 56: Are breastfeeding problems related to incorrect breastfeeding technique and the use of pacifiers and bottles?

Method: Case-control study

Authors	Date	Where published	Intervention assessed	Entry criteria	Number of women studied	Outcomes measured	Results
Righard L	1998	Birth 25 (1): 40–44	Evaluation of the involvement of incorrect breastfeeding technique and the use of pacifiers and bottles on breastfeeding problems	Healthy mother-infant pairs attending hospital-based outpatient clinic and local child health clinics in Malmö, Sweden	92 healthy mother-infant pairs	Prevalence of 'incorrect sucking technique'	94% among cases, compared with 10% among controls (p=0.0001)
					52 cases referred to outpatient clinic with problems of breastfeeding	Prevalence of pacifier use	73% among cases, versus 30% among controls (p=0.003)
							73% of pacifier users had a 'superficial sucking technique', compared with 41% of non-pacifier users (p=0.016)
				Multiple problems were reported by cases, 3 most frequent were: baby restless or crying during or between feeds (62%), sore nipples (33%), concerns for adequate nutrition leading to introduction of supplementary bottles (23%)	40 controls attending community-based child health clinics for routine baby check-ups	Breastfeeding outcome as a function of supplementary bottle use	31% of mothers (6/19) who had introduced bottles before referral had stopped breastfeeding at clinic follow-up, compared with 6% (2/33) of those who had not introduced bottles at time of referral (p=0.04)
						Differences between cases and controls	*No significant differences in maternal age, marital status, coffee drinking or smoking. Significantly more primiparous women among cases (73%), than among controls (47%) (p<0.05)*

TABLE 57: Do infant formula samples shorten the duration of breastfeeding?

Method: A randomised controlled trial

Authors	Date	Where published	Intervention assessed	Entry criteria	Number of women studied	Outcomes measured	Results
Bergevin Y Dougherty C Kramer MS	1983	Lancet i: 1148–1151	Provision of a formula sample versus no formula sample	Breastfeeding women	406 212 were given a formula sample 194 had no formula sample	Duration of breastfeeding	78% of mothers who had received a sample were breastfeeding at 1 month compared with 84% of mothers who had no sample (p=0.07) 67% of women who had less than 14 years of education and had received a sample were breastfeeding at 1 month compared with 79% of this group of women who had not received a sample
						Introduction of supplementary formula	47 (22%) of those women who had been given a formula sample, were giving 1 or more bottles of formula a day at 4–6 weeks postpartum compared with 31 (16%) of those women who had not received a sample

TABLE 58: Commercial discharge packs and breastfeeding counselling: effects on infant feeding practices in a randomised trial

Method: Randomised trial

Authors	Date	Where published	Intervention assessed	Entry criteria	Number of women studied	Outcomes measured	Results
Frank DA Wirtz SJ Sorenson JR Heeren T	1987	Paediatrics 80(6): 845–854	There were two interventions: 1. Routine breast-feeding advice; this consisted of a discharge teaching session covering all aspects of baby care and included some information on breastfeeding, this varied from nurse to nurse versus Research breastfeeding counselling; this was a 20–40 minute research based information giving session with a trained counsellor, followed by 8 pre-arranged telephone calls from the counsellor between 5 days and 12 weeks postpartum 2. Commercial discharge packs containing free bottle/water samples versus Research discharge packs containing educational materials and breastpads	Women having breastfed at least once in hospital; English or Spanish speakers; with a telephone available at home; with a healthy infant with no more than 48 hours neonatal care required	324	Duration of breastfeeding	Percentage of women exclusively breastfeeding Routine breastfeeding counselling and commercial discharge pack (n=83) Infants age (months) 1 2 3 4 53% 20% 6% 5% Routine breastfeeding counselling and research discharge pack (n=78) Infants age (months) 1 2 3 4 53% 28% 15% 6% Research breastfeeding counselling and commercial discharge pack (n=84) Infants age (months) 1 2 3 4 57% 29% 6% 2% Research breastfeeding counselling and research discharge pack (n=79) Infants age (months) 1 2 3 4 62% 43% 20% 9% Significant effects of both interventions at 2 months (packs p=0.014, counselling p=0.005) and for discharge packs at 3 months (p=0.0005) and 4 months (p=0.035)

TABLE 59: The effect of infant formula samples on breastfeeding practice

Method: Randomised trial

Authors	Date	Where published	Intervention assessed	Entry criteria	Number of women studied	Outcomes measured	Results
Evans CJ Lyons NB Killien MG	1986	JOGNN 15: 401–405	Provision of formula sample versus no formula sample Women were randomised using 'slips of paper'	Women who were breastfeeding their babies Mother and baby discharged together	95 No formula sample group = 40 Formula sample group = 55	Duration of breastfeeding	There was no statistical difference in the number of babies bottle fed at 6 weeks between the two groups

TABLE 60: Factors related to early termination of breastfeeding in an urban population

Method: A double-blind randomised study

Authors	Date	Where published	Intervention assessed	Entry criteria	Number of women studied	Outcomes measured	Results	
Feinstein JM Berkelhamer JE Gruszka ME Wong CA Carey AE	1986	Paediatrics 78(2): 210–215	Provision of formula samples versus No formula samples	Women who were planning to breastfeed	166 Discharge pack with formula group n=76 Discharge pack without formula group n=90	Duration of breastfeeding	Formula group	No formula group
						Breastfeeding at 1 month	64/76 (84%)	79/90 (88%)
						Breastfeeding at 10 weeks	55/76 (72%)	65/90 (72%)
						Breastfeeding at 4 months	44/76 (58%)	50/90 (56%)
						Type of breastfeeding at 1 month		
						Fully breastfeeding	42/76 (55%)	49/90 (54%)
						Partial breastfeeding	19/76 (28%)	25/90 (28%)

TABLE 61: Effect of discharge samples on duration of breast-feeding

Method: Randomised trial

Authors	Date	Where published	Intervention assessed	Entry criteria	Number of women studied	Outcomes measured	Results
Dungy CI Christensen-Szalanski J Losch M Russell D	1992	Pediatrics 90:2: 233–237	Provision of discharge packs containing an infant formula versus a pack containing a manual breast pump	USA: Healthy mothers either exclusively breastfeeding or breast and formula feeding	146 A high attrition rate of approx 40%, only follow up data on 87 mothers	Duration exclusive breastfeeding At 2 weeks: At 4 weeks: At 6 weeks: At 8 weeks:	Packs with formula (n=43) 23 women (53.5%) were exclusively breastfeeding Packs with pump (n=44) 32 women (72.7%) were exclusively breastfeeding Packs with formula (n=43) 15 women (34.9%) were exclusively breastfeeding Packs with pump (n=44) 24 women (54.5%) were exclusively breastfeeding Packs with formula (n=43) 13 women (30.2%) were exclusively breastfeeding Packs with pump (n=44) 20 women (45.5%) were exclusively breastfeeding Packs with formula (n=43) 10 women (23.3%) were exclusively breastfeeding Packs with pump (n=44) 16 women (36.4%) were exclusively breastfeeding

TABLE 62: The association of formula samples given at hospital dicharged with the early duration of breastfeeding

Method: Randomised trial

Authors	Date	Where published	Intervention assessed	Entry criteria	Number of women studied	Outcomes measured	Results
Snell B J Krantz M Keeton R Delgado K Peckham C	1992	J Hum Lact 8(2): 67–72	Provision of a gift pack containing a sample of infant formula (control) versus not receiving a gift pack (experimental group)	Hispanic women in USA (lower socio-economic status), all breastfeeding with a healthy full-term newborn, and all having a telephone Spanish speaking group who traditionally use water and tea as routine 'medicinal' supplements	88 38 received a gift pack containing formula (GP group) 50 received no gift pack (NGP group)	Feeding practices At 1 week: At 3 weeks: 33 responders in GP group, 47 in NGP group	68% of women in the Gift Pack group (GP) compared with 80% in the No GP group (NGP) were breastfeeding exclusively, although this difference was not significant. Similarly, 3% (n=1) compared with 6% (n=3) were bottle-feeding (n.s.) 33% of women in the GP group were breastfeeding exclusively, compared with 68% in the NGP group (p<0.004). 27% of women in the GP group had switched to bottle-feeding compared with 13% in the NGP group

TABLE 63: The effect of discharge pack formula and breast pumps on breastfeeding duration and choice of infant feeding method

Method: Randomised trial

Authors	Date	Where published	Intervention assessed	Entry criteria	Number of women studied	Outcomes measured	Results

Bliss M C
Wilkie J
Acredolo C
Berman S
Tebb K P
	1997	Birth 24(2): 90–101	Giving discharge packs containing either infant formula, a manual breast pump, both or neither	All English-speaking women (with a telephone) delivering in a 13 month period. Babies deemed to be at low risk and to have no complications
				
				1,625 women recruited through information sheet/consent form, from total births of 6,350 (26%)
				
				Hospital has Certificate of Intent under BFHI
					1,625 assigned at random to four groups:
					
					Group A: Neither formula sample nor breast pump added to pack
					
					Group B: Manual breast pump included in pack
					
					Group C: Can of powdered infant formula in pack
					
					Group D: Both infant formula and breast pump included in pack
						Fully or partially breastfeeding, or formula feeding at:
						6 weeks
						
						4 months
						
						6 months
						
						Mean weeks breastfed
							%Full %Partial %Formula
							Group A 54.4 24.4 21.1
							Group B 57.3 20.8 22.0
							Group C 52.6 28.9 18.6
							Group D 52.2 24.7 23.1
							Differences not significant
							
							      %Full %Partial %Formula
							Group A 35.6 15.3 49.1
							Group B 35.0 19.6 45.4
							Group C 34.7 21.7 43.6
							Group D 31.0 19.0 15.1
							Differences not significant
							
							      %Full %Partial %Formula
							Group A 23.9 12.7 63.4
							Group B 23.3 15.2 61.6
							Group C 23.3 19.3 57.4
							Group D 19.2 15.1 65.7
							Differences not significant
							
							      Mean weeks:
							Group A 15.7 wks
							Group B 16.0 wks
							Group C 16.7 wks
							Group D 15.7 wks
							Differences not significant

TABLE 64: Hospital infant formula discharge packages

Method: Randomised trial

Authors	Date	Where published	Intervention assessed	Entry criteria	Number of women studied	Outcomes measured	Results
Dungy C I Losch M E Russell D Romitti P Dusdieker L B	1997	Arch Paediatr Adolesc Med 151: 724–29	Providing discharge packs containing either: 1. a manual breast pump (m.b.p.) 2. a sample of infant formula (i.f.s.), or 3. both a manual breast and infant formula samples (m.b.p.+ i.f.s.)	All women delivering in a single maternity unit over a twelve month period, who agreed to participate (810/1012) N.B. *Rates of exclusive breastfeeding were 30% higher on average than rates in the previous study of Dungy et al (1992) showing a negative impact of discharge packs*	763	Percentage of women in each group reporting exclusive or partial breastfeeding during 16 week follow-up Mean duration (weeks) of exclusive and partial breastfeeding	Exclusive Partial Group 1 (m.b.p.) 16.7% 37.1% Group 2 (i.f.s.) 16.3% 33.8% Group 3 (m.b.p.+i.f.s.) 18.4% 33.9% These differences not significant, although time-survival analysis indicated that women in group 3 showed a higher rate of exclusive breastfeeding through weeks 2 to 8 (p<0.01) after controlling for other variables Exclusive Partial Group 1 (m.b.p.) 6.13±0.39 10.03±0.38 Group 2 (i.f.s.) 7.10±0.37 10.21±0.36 Group 3 (m.b.p.+i.f.s.) 6.43±0.38 9.79±0.37 Differences not significant

TABLE 65: Effect of two types of hospital feeding gift packs on duration of breastfeeding among adolescent mothers

Method: A randomised prospective study

Authors	Date	Where published	Intervention assessed	Entry criteria	Number of women studied	Outcomes measured	Results
Neifert M Gray J Camp B	1988	Journal of Adolescent Health Care 9: 411–413	A commercial breast-feeding gift pack that contained formula versus a gift pack with breastfeeding aids but without formula	Adolescent mothers <18 yrs of age – primiparous, breastfeeding a healthy baby weighing >2500 g Breastfed at least once following delivery	60	Duration of breastfeeding Age at which formula supplementation was introduced	No data were provided indicating the relative incidence of the outcomes by treatment group The authors report no significant differences in either of the outcome measures Overall: 35% of the entire group of 60 women breastfed for less than 1 month, and 43% for more than 2 months. the remaining 22% breastfed between 1–2 months

TABLE 66: Effect of a traditional and of a new nipple shield on sucking patterns and milk flow

Method: Comparison study

Authors	Date	Where published	Intervention assessed	Entry criteria	Number of women studied	Outcomes measured	Results
Woolridge M Baum J Drewett R	1980	Early Human Development 4(4): 357–364	Comparison study between 'Mexican Hat' nipple shield and thin latex nipple shield	Breastfeeding with no problems 5–8 days postpartum	34 16 mothers using 'Mexican Hat' nipple shield 18 mothers using latex nipple shield	Milk transfer at a feed Sucking patterns	Amount significantly reduced with 'Mexican Hat', from 46.4 g (normal) to 19.5 g (with Mexican Hat) (p<0.01) Difference in mean milk intake with thin latex shield not significant; 38.4 g (normal) to 29.9 g (with shield) Sucking rate (within a burst) faster with 'Mexican Hat' (p<0.05), and more time spent pausing (p<0.01) Differences in sucking pattern with thin latex nipple shield not significant

TABLE 67: The effect of nipple shields on maternal milk volume: study with alternating treatments

Method: Non-randomised, prospective comparison study

Authors	Date	Where published	Intervention assessed	Entry criteria	Number of women studied	Outcomes measured	Results
Auerbach KG	1990	JOGNN 19(5): 419–427	The effect of two designs of nipple shield on pumped milk volume compared with pumped milk volume without nipple shield Each woman was her own control	Lactation well established Babies thriving Mothers using or planning to use the University of Chicago Lactation Station to pump their breast milk on their return to work	25	Volume of milk obtained Differences in milk volume by nipple shield used	Compared with no shield, x4 amount obtained with new shield x6 amount obtained with old shield No significant difference The author identifies five questions the nurse should ask before suggesting the use of a nipple shield

TABLE 68: Cracked nipples in breastfeeding mothers

Method: Randomised trial

Authors	Date	Where published	Intervention assessed	Entry criteria	Number of women studied	Outcomes measured	Results
Nicholson W	1985	Nursing Mothers Association of Australia 21(4): 7–10	Women who developed a cracked nipple were randomly assigned to one of three groups 1. Discontinuation of breastfeeding with expression of milk from the affected breast until the nipple healed 2. The use of a nipple shield on the affected breast until the nipple healed 3. Continued breastfeeding on the affected side with supervision and help	Mothers who developed a cracked nipple	90 30 women in each group	Nipple healed Duration of breastfeeding Adherence to treatment Appearance of new cracks in nipples	26 (87%) of the nipples in Group 1 healed 26 (87%) of the nipples in Group 2 healed 23 (77%) of the nipples in Group 3 healed 4 women in Group 1 stopped breastfeeding 1 woman in Group 2 stopped breastfeeding No women in Group 3 stopped breastfeeding 24(80%) of women in Group 1 adhered to treatment 8 (27%) of women in Group 2 adhered to treatment 21(70%) of women in Group 3 adhered to treatment 1 crack appeared in Group 1 4 cracks appeared in Group 2 no cracks appeared in Group 3

TABLE 69: The use of nipple shields by breastfeeding women

Method: Descriptive study

Authors	Date	Where published	Method	Entry criteria	Number of women studied	Outcomes measured	Results
Nicholson W	1993	Australian College of Midwives Incorporated Journal 6(2): 18–24	Descriptive case study on women using nipple shields for their breastfeeding problem, and on women not recommended to use nipple shields Survey sample of breastfeeding women who were not seen by the lactation consultant postnatally	Incidental sample of breastfeeding women during 1988–1989 seen by the lactation consultant by request from postnatal midwives because the women had breastfeeding problems	822 women who saw a lactation consultant Of these 186 women used nipple shields (NS), and 636 women did not use nipple shields (NN) 349 in post natal group who did not see the lactation consultant (PN)	Breastfeeding on discharge Breastfeeding at 3 months Problems reported at 3 months Patients still using nipple shield at 3 months	NS: 176/186 (95%) NN: 530/636 (83%) PN: 318/349 (91%) (NS versus NN p<0.001) (NN versus PN p<0.001) NS: 92/166 (55%) of women contacted were breastfeeding, 84/166 (51%) exclusively NN: 298/473 (63%) of women contacted were breastfeeding, 256/473 (54%) exclusively PN: 190/282 (67%) of women contacted were breastfeeding, 161/282 (57%) exclusively (NS versus PN p=0.01) Nipple trauma: NS: 15/166 (9%) NN: 27/473 (6%) PN: 19/282 (7%) Mastitis: NS: 20/166 (12%) NN: 40/473 (8%) PN: 19/282 (7%) Breastfeeding with nipple shield = 13/92 (14%)

TABLE 70: Effect of a breast shell on postpartum nipple pain

Method: Non-randomised prospective comparison study

Authors	Date	Where published	Intervention assessed	Entry criteria	Number of women studied	Outcomes measured	Results
Gosha JL Tichy AM	1988	Journal of Nurse-Midwifery 33(2): 74–77	Effect of a breast shell in the treatment of postpartum nipple pain: 1. Inserting a breast shell over one nipple 2. No treatment of the other nipple	Breastfeeding women who were experiencing nipple pain in the first week postpartum	Convenience sample of 20 women	Nipple pain	No significant difference was found in the levels of pain between the nipple treated with a shell and the untreated nipple

TABLE 71: Evaluation of a Dressing to Reduce Nipple Pain and Improve Nipple Skin Condition in Breastfeeding Women

Method: Prospective comparison study

Authors	Date	Where published	Intervention assessed	Entry criteria	Number of women studied	Outcomes measured	Results
Ziemer MM Cooper DM Pigeon JG	1995	Nursing Research 44(6): 347–351	Women applied a polyethylene film dressing with a perimeter adhesive system to a randomly determined nipple for 7 days. The other nipple acted as the control. The dressing was removed prior to feeds and replaced immediately after	White women who had had uncomplicated deliveries. Had not been lactating in the previous 12 months	50. 26 women dropped out of the study but were replaced	1. Incidence of erythema, blisters, fissures and oedema 2. Nipple pain 3. Comfort of the dressing	No significant differences were found in the erythema intensity, occurrence of blisters, fissures or oedema between the treated and untreated nipple. Significant differences in the pain scores (p<.05) Average pain ratings: treated nipple = 1.48 untreated nipple = 1.76. Most women (66%) found removal of the dressing uncomfortable. 77% of the women experienced a rash on the area of the skin in contact with the perimeter adhesive system

TABLE 72: Twenty cases of persistent sore nipples. Collaboration between consultant and dermatologist

Method: Case studies

Authors	Date	Where published	Method	Entry criteria	Number of women studied	Outcomes measured	Results
Huggins KE Billon SF	1993	J Hum Lact 9(3): 155–60	The lactation consultant referred women with continuing nipple pain to a dermatologist. The dermatologist saw the referred women 2–3 days following referral. Various treatments were given: Topical steroids Topical antibiotics	Mothers with continuing nipple pain	20	Continued nipple pain or improved.	18 out of the 20 women referred showed improvement

TABLE 73: Effect of the method of breastfeeding on breast engorgement, mastitis and infantile colic

Method: Non-randomised comparison study

Authors	Date	Where published	Intervention assessed	Entry criteria	Number of women studied	Outcomes measured	Results
Evans K Evans R Simmer K	1995	Acta Paediatrica 84: 849–52	Comparison of two methods of breastfeeding on breast engorgement 1. Experimental group: prolonged emptying of one breast at each feed 2. Control group: both breasts drained equally at each feed	Breastfeeding women	Total 302 Experimental group n=150 Control group n=152	Incidence of engorgement Mastitis Infantile colic	There was significantly less engorgement in the experimental group: 61.4% in experimental group 74% in control group (p<0.02) There was no significant difference in the incidence of mastitis Significant difference: 12% in experimental 23% in control (p<0.02) Only one-third (43) of mothers in the experimental group felt that one breast satisfied the infant's hunger and the others offered the second breast at the end of the feed

TABLE 74: Ultrasound treatment for breast engorgement

Method: Double blind randomised controlled trial

Authors	Date	Where published	Intervention assessed	Entry criteria	Number of women studied	Outcomes measured	Results
McLachlan Z Milne EJ Lumley J Walker BL	1991	Australian Journal of Physiotherapy 37: 23–29	Effect of ultrasound energy on engorgement Two ultrasound machines, one without the ultrasonic crystal Each breast referred was randomized to either treatment A or B before and following treatment Visual analogue scales for pain and hardness were completed for each breast	Referral to physiotherapist for treatment of breast engorgement Excluded were women who had previously received breast implants (silicone)	197 breasts	Pain and hardness; comparison between ultrasound and sham treated breasts	No significant difference between breast treated with either sham or ultrasound was found in either pain or hardness, but both treatments helped Components which might have contributed to the therapeutic effect: warmth, rest, massage, attention, and the emotional, practical, and informational support provided by the physiotherapists during treatment

TABLE 75: Do cabbage leaves prevent breast engorgement?

Method: Randomised controlled trial

Authors	Date	Where published	Intervention assessed	Entry criteria	Number of women studied	Outcomes measured	Results
Nikodem VC Danziger D Gebka N Gulmezoglu A Hofmeyr GJ	1993	Birth 20: 61–64	Cabbage leaf application to the breasts versus routine care	Breastfeeding women	120 breastfeeding women 60 in experimental group 60 in control group	1. Maternal perception of engorgement following application of cabbage leaves 2. Time intervals between feeds 3. Duration of breastfeeding post-delivery	No significant effect on engorgement between the two groups There was no significant difference between the two groups Fewer mothers in the experimental group stopped breastfeeding before 8 days. Slightly more mothers in the experimental group were exclusively breastfeeding at the 6-week follow up

TABLE 76: A comparison of chilled cabbage leaves and chilled gel packs in reducing breast engorgement

Method: Non-randomised prospective comparison study

Authors	Date	Where published	Intervention assessed	Entry criteria	Number of women studied	Outcomes measured	Results
Roberts KL	1995	J Hum Lact 11(1): 17–20	Non-random treatment assignment was used Women with an even hospital registration number were given a gelpak to use on their right breast and chilled cabbage leaves to use on their left breast Women with an odd hospital registration number were given the opposite One pre treatment pain measurement and two post treatment measurements, one for each breast	Non-aboriginal, lactating women with breast engorgement, in this case engorgement was summarised as hard, warm painful breasts, with difficulty breastfeeding	34	Relief of breast engorgement	There were no statistically significant differences in either the time of the onset of relief for the two treatments or in the effect of the treatments There was a statistically significant reduction of pain achieved by both treatments

TABLE 77: A comparison of chilled and room temperature cabbage leaves in treating breast engorgement

Method: Non-randomised prospective comparison study

Authors	Date	Where published	Intervention assessed	Entry criteria	Number of women studied	Outcomes measured	Results
Roberts KL Reiter M Schuster D	1995	J Hum Lact 11(3): 191–194	Mothers were assigned to treatment groups: One had chilled cabbage leaves on the right breast and room temperature cabbage leaves on the left Other treatment group were reversed No control One pre-treatment pain measurement Two post-treatment pain measurements	Convenience sample of 28 lactating inpatient women from two hospitals in Darwin Lactation and engorgement	28	Day engorgement began Results of treatment	Day 2: 36% Day 3: 36% Day 4 or later: 28% 70% experienced difficulty in feeding due to engorgement No significant difference between chilled or room temperature cabbage leaves; both were associated with a significant reported reduction in pain

TABLE 78: The clinical effects of 'protease complex' on postpartum breast engorgement

Method: Double blind randomised controlled trial

Authors	Date	Where published	Intervention assessed	Entry criteria	Number of women studied	Outcomes measured	Results
Murata T Hunzow M Nomura Y	1965	J Jap Obstet Gynecol Soc 12(3): 139–147	Oral protease (20,000 units bomelain and 2500 units crystalline trypsin) versus placebo Both groups, 2 tablets q.d.s. on day 1 On days 2 and 3, 1 tablet q.d.s. 16 tablets in total	Breastfeeding women in hospital Symptoms of engorgement on 3rd to 5th day post-partum Complaints of pain and tenderness rated on a 4-point scale	59 women 35 in experimental group 24 in control group	Observed effect on breast engorgement	29/35 (83%) women in experimental group reported improvement in engorgement 6/35 (17%) showed no change in engorgement; no cases worse 8/24 (33%) women in control group reported improvement in engorgement 14/24 (58%) reported no change in engorgement 2/24 (8%) cases worse Significant differences between experimental and control groups (p<0.05)

TABLE 79: The treatment of breast engorgement with serrapeptase (Danzen)

Method: Randomised double blind trial

Authors	Date	Where published	Intervention assessed	Entry criteria	Number of women studied	Outcomes measured	Results
Kee WH Tan SL Lee V Salmon YM	1989	Singapore Med Jnl 30(1): 48–54	Oral Danzen versus placebo 2 tablets x 3 daily x 3 days	Women diagnosed as suffering breast engorgement, defined as: subjective complaint of pain in the breast and objective evidence of breast swelling, induration and impaired lactation.	70 Experimental group n=35 women Control group n=35 women	Degree of breast engorgement Degree of breast swelling Breast pain	Experimental group: 30 (85%) showed a moderate to marked improvement following Danzen treatment Control group: 21 (60%) showed a moderate to marked improvement following treatment with placebo Experimental group: 26 (74%) showed a moderate to marked improvement following Danzen treatment Control group: 23 (65%) showed a moderate to marked improvement following treatment with placebo Experimental group: 30 (85%) showed a moderate to marked improvement following Danzen treatment Control group: 26 (74%) showed a moderate to marked improvement following treatment with placebo

TABLE 80: Mastitis today: incidence, prevention and treatment

Method: Survey

Authors	Date	Where published	Method	Entry criteria	Number of women studied	Outcomes measured	Results
Jonsson S Pulkkinen MO	1994	Annales Chirurgiae et Gynaecologiae 83: 84–87	Questionnaire 5–12 weeks postpartum Of those who answered the questionnaire, 255 women chosen 'at random' were advised to do breast massage with the hand, a brush, a coarse towel, or a sponge before and/or after delivery	Answered the questionnaire in one of 24 outpatient clinics	664	Overall frequency of mastitis	24% of the 664 women reported an episode of mastitis (among these 10.4% had stopped breastfeeding) Of 329 multiparous women, 80 had mastitis. Of those, 54% had had mastitis during the previous puerperium. Probability of subsequent mastitis is threefold (p=0.007). Mothers under 21 and over 33 had lowered incidence (p=0.034)
						Factors associated with incidence of mastitis	Skin type, reaction to sun, allergies, rashes, getting cold and oxytocin during delivery did not affect the incidence. 201 women had sore nipples of whom 30.8% had an episode of mastitis. This did not affect the incidence
						Incidence of mastitis in the 255 women who had been given advice	In 38% of mastitis episodes antibiotics were used Women who used nipple cream several times a day or even only a few times a month had an increased incidence of mastitis (p=0.001)

TABLE 81: Mastitis among lactating women occurrence and risk factors

Method: Retrospective cohort study

Authors	Date	Where published	Method	Entry criteria	Number of women studied	Outcomes measured	Results
Kaufmann R Foxman B	1991	Social Science and Medicine 33(6): 701–705	This was a historical cohort study which investigated the incidence and timing of sporadic puerperal mastitis, data was collected from the delivery and post-natal follow-up records	Gave birth at the study hospital between 1984 and 1985 Seen prenatally at obstetrics and gynaecology clinic Breastfeeding at discharge	966 lactating women	Mastitis in the first 7 weeks postpartum, diagnosed by or reported to hospital	2.9% Associated with: - employed mother - 2 professional parents - older mother - birth in 'delivery room' rather than in 'labour room' Not associated with parity

TABLE 82: A descriptive study of lactation mastitis in long-term breastfeeding women

Method: Survey

Authors	Date	Where published	Method	Entry criteria	Number of women studied	Outcomes measured	Results
Riordan JM Nicholls FH	1990	J Hum Lact 6(2): 53–58	Collected descriptive data on the experience of mastitis from breastfeeding mothers Phase 1: A questionnaire was handed out at a conference Phase 2: A follow-up questionnaire 6 months after the first survey	Three groups of participants at conferences sponsored by the International Lactation Consultants Association Almost all breastfed more than one infant for several months or longer	91	1. The incidence of mastitis among long-term breastfeeding women 2. Factors associated with the development of mastitis 3. Treatment breastfeeding women use to resolve mastitis 4. Whether mastitis is likely to occur more in one area of the breast than others	33% of entire sample reported at least one episode. Mean: 2.1 Fatigue 24% Stress 22% Plugged duct 17% 54% of women with mastitis had antibiotic treatment Upper outer quadrant of the breast was found to be most frequent site of infection Limitations: group surveyed were more knowledgeable about mastitis than the average population

TABLE 83: Breastfeeding practices and lactational mastitis

Method: Survey and case control study

Authors	Date	Where published	Method	Entry criteria	Number of women studied	Outcomes measured	Results
Foxman B Schwarz K Looman S	1994	Social Science and Medicine 38(5): 755–761	1. 100 women were surveyed 2. 17 matched pairs both cases and controls answered a questionnaire which was delivered in 30-minute telephone interview	Study participants were recruited from an early discharge programme for two hospitals 9 mastitis cases identified from survey and 8 women who did not complete questionnaire referred by clinic staff Control then selected from these	100 survey 17 matched pairs = 34	Characteristics of study population participating in breastfeeding survey Breastfeeding practices Characteristics of mastitis cases and controls	100 women. Mean age 30 97% white 96% married 45% first experience of breastfeeding 54% Bachelor's degree 69% experienced engorgement in the first week 74% nipple pain 89% used the 'Madonna position' 63% changed breast during feeds Mastitis occurred most commonly in the first 6 weeks postpartum 82% had pain in the breast or nipple in the week prior to mastitis Only 41% of mastitis cases regularly had a rest during the day compared with 70.6% of controls

TABLE 84: Mastitis: infection or inflammation?

Method: Observational study

Authors	Date	Where published	Method	Entry criteria	Number of women studied	Outcomes measured	Results
Inch S Fisher C	1995	Practitioner 239: 472–476	Tested the null hypothesis that there is no relationship between the side affected with mastitis and the preferred holding side by comparing preferred holding side with side on which breast affected	All women presenting to the breastfeeding clinic with mastitis	77	Relationship between the side affected with mastitis and the women's handedness	Unclear in ten cases In 49 women (78%) the mastitis had developed in the breast opposite the preferred holding side In 14 women (22%) the mastitis had developed on the same side The null hypothesis was rejected with over 99.5% confidence

TABLE 85: Acute puerperal mastitis: evaluation of its management

Method: Retrospective description of care management

Authors	Date	Where published	Intervention assessed	Entry criteria	Number of women studied	Outcomes measured	Results
Devereux WP	1969	Amer J Obstet 108(1): 78–81	Early simple support - intermittent cold pack - continual nursing - analgesics - Sulfisoxazole q.d.s. 5/7 - occasionally, other antibiotics	In the author's private practice 1948–1968 With endemic [not hospital-acquired epidemic] infection] (>101°) acute febrile mastitis (swollen, pink area of breast)	53 (71 episodes)	Continued lactation Abscesses Infant illness attributable to continued breastfeeding with mastitis	Lactation and nursing continued in 47 cases. It is unclear whether this is 47/53 or 47/71 In 8 (11.1%) of 9 instances when treatment was delayed longer than 24 hours, 6 developed abscesses None N.B. Abscess was considered a strict contra-indication to breastfeeding

TABLE 86: Course and treatment of milk stasis, non-infectious inflammation of the breast, and infectious mastitis in nursing women

Method: Randomised controlled trial

Authors	Date	Where published	Intervention assessed	Entry criteria	Number of women studied	Outcomes measured	Results
Thomsen AC Espersen T Maigaard S	1984	Amer J Obstet Gynaecol 1499(5): 492–495	Differential diagnosis based on Leucocyte counts of the milk and quantitative cultivations for bacteria Within each diagnostic group, women randomly allocated to non-intervention or treatment. Treatment involved breast emptying and in some cases, antibiotics	Not given Method of randomisation not given	213 (339 inflamed breasts) 126 with milk stasis 48 with non-infectious inflammation 110 with infectious mastitis	Duration and outcome of milk stasis, non-infectious inflammation and infectious mastitis	Regular breast emptying improved outcome in all groups Recurrence of infection and abscesses (6 cases) was only in the infectious mastitis without treatment group *Staph. aureus* isolated from all cases of abscess

TABLE 87: Infant insufficient milk syndrome associated with maternal postpartum haemorrhage

Method: Case studies

Authors	Date	Where published	Results
Willis CE Livingstone V	1995	J Hum Lact 11: 123–126	10 consecutive cases Mothers who had postpartum haemorrhage, whose babies had insufficient milk intake Attending large breastfeeding referral clinic One case described, the others in a table They postulate, "PPH can produce a transient hypotensive insult and temporary pituitary ischaemia which inhibits the hormonal triggering of lactogenesis II by prolactin." They recommend further investigation of any baby with weight loss >7% of birthweight

TABLE 88: Anemia and insufficient milk in first-time mothers

Method: Longitudinal study

Authors	Date	Where published	Method	Entry criteria	Number of women studied	Outcomes measured	Results
Henly SJ Anderson CM Avery MD Hills-Bonczyk SG Potter S Duckett LJ	1995	Birth 22: 87–92	Women completed questionnaires prior to discharge Postpartum haemoglobin was taken from the women's' notes Women were re-contacted by telephone at 1, 3, 6, 9, and 12 months Questionnaire re-weaning was sent to the mothers Haemoglobin of <10.0 g/dl was classified as anemic	Breastfeeding Primiparous From one large urban private hospital in north-central USA Above 18 years Speaks, reads, and writes English	630	Anemia <10.0 g/dl haemoglobin Insufficient milk syndrome Duration of breastfeeding Age at weaning and reason for weaning	137 women (22%) had haemoglobin levels <10.0 g/dl The percentage of women reporting insufficient milk syndrome was greater for those with anemia (19.7%) than those without (11.4%) Both duration and the infant age at weaning were significantly shorter for the women with the syndrome Women reporting insufficient milk breastfed fully for a mean rate of 3.8 weeks. The infant weaning mean rate for women reporting insufficient milk was 12.1 weeks Women without insufficient milk breastfed fully for a mean rate of 3.8 weeks. The infant weaning mean rate for women without insufficient milk was 30.7 weeks

TABLE 89: The influence of breast surgery, breast appearance, pregnancy-induced breast changes on lactation sufficiency as measured by infant weight gain

Method: Prospective study

Authors	Date	Where published	Method	Entry criteria	Number of women studied	Outcomes measured	Results
Neifert M de Marzo S Seacat J Young D Leff M Orleans M	1990	Birth 17: 31–38	Postpartum visits: 1. 4–7 days breasts photographed 2. 9–14 days Advice on nursing technique, advice on frequency of feeds	Healthy women Motivated Primiparous Breastfeeding Term babies	319	Lactation outcome Previous breast surgery Prenatal breast size and pregnancy-induced breast changes Postpartum breast enlargement with engorgement Breast symmetry Nipple protuberance	Within 3 weeks postpartum 85% of mothers achieved sufficient lactation 6.9% had undergone breast surgery Women with periareolar breast incisions were five times more likely to experience lactation insufficiency Women with insufficient lactation significantly more likely to report only minimal (none or only slight) breast enlargement Lactation outcome did not differ significantly for women with asymmetries Lactation outcome did not differ significantly for women with flat nipples in this study

TABLE 90: Factors affecting the duration of breastfeeding: 2. Early feeding practices and social class

Method: Observation study

Authors	Date	Where published	Method	Entry criteria	Number of women studied	Outcomes measured	Results
Houston MJ Howie PW Smart L McArdle T McNeilly AS	1983	Early Human Development 55–63	Babies' breast milk intake measured by test-weighing on 3rd and 6th postpartum day Mothers' home environment assessed by social class Information about feeds obtained by charts	Breastfeeding Birthweight >2500 g Gestation >38 weeks Progressing normally and not jaundiced on the 3rd day Mothers resident in Edinburgh On postnatal ward at Simpson Memorial Maternity Pavilion during 4-week recruitment period	47	Breastmilk intake measured by test weighing on the 3rd postpartum day Duration of breastfeeding 6th day test-weigh Baby weight Number of breastfeeds Time of first feed Volume of extra fluid Social class	High milk transfer = >200 g/day (n=13) Medium milk transfer = 50–200 g/day (n=22) Low milk transfer = <50 g/day (n=12) Women with low milk transfer were significantly more likely to have stopped breastfeeding by 6 weeks Significant differences in intake between high, medium and low groups Weight loss significantly less on day 6 in the infants in the high milk transfer group Significantly more feeds in the high milk transfer group No significant difference Less to 'high' group. Significant difference from day 4 Longer breastfeeding with higher social class Significant difference at 6 and 16 weeks

TABLE 91: The effect of maternal fluid intake on breast milk supply: a pilot study

Method: Pilot study and cross-over design

Authors	Date	Where published	Intervention assessed	Entry criteria	Number of women studied	Outcomes measured	Results
Morse JM Ewing G Gamble D Donahue P	1992	Canadian Journal of Public Health 213–216	3 days of normal fluid intake (based on body weight, not thirst)	Mothers had breastfed previously	10 mother-baby pairs	Milk supply (determined by test-weighing and measuring leaked milk)	Milk supply up with fluids and down with fluids, but not significant
			3 days of fluid intake 50% greater than normal	Normal delivery			
			3 days of fluid intake 50% less than normal (this was close to what women usually drank)	Married			
				22–35 years old			
				Healthy			
				Non-smokers			
				Not employed			
				Tertiary education			
				Breastfed at discrete intervals throughout the day			

TABLE 92: Prolactin, fluid balance and lactation

Method: Non randomised intervention study

Authors	Date	Where published	Intervention assessed	Entry criteria	Number of women studied	Outcomes measured	Results
Dearlove JC Dearlove BM	1981	Brit J Obstet Gynaecol 88: 652–654	Performed on day 6 or 7 from the onset of lactation Each women fasted overnight Then drank 20 ml of water per kilo of body weight Serum prolactin and milk yield measured	Healthy non-smoking women in their second successful lactation	Not stated	Mean serum prolactin Mean serum osmolarity Mean breast milk yield Mean osmolarity	No change Reduced No change No change Recommends: Thirst should regulate fluid intake. The practice of encouraging lactating women to drink excessively should be discontinued

TABLE 93: Lactation failure

Method: Non-randomised, uncontrolled study

Authors	Date	Where published	Method	Entry criteria	Number of women studied	Outcomes measured	Results
Mathur GP Chitranshi S Mathur S Singh SB Bhalla M	1992	Indian Pediatrics 29(12): 309–15	Relactation was attempted in all cases Mothers were given rest, nutrition and psychological support Frequent and prolonged sucking by the baby fixed in the correct position If lactation was not established Maxalon 10mg was given 8-hourly for 10 days	75 mothers whose <4 month old infants were admitted to the authors' hospital, Kanphr Medical College The infants were ill and the mothers were diagnosed to have either complete or partial lactation failure	75	Rate of relactation Demographic details	Of the women studied, 71 (94.7%) had partial lactation failure. Following treatment 49 (69.3%) women successfully relactated 4 (5.3%) of the women studied had complete failure Relactation was successful in 3 (75%) of those cases 56% of the women delivered in hospital 44% at home 86% of the women received antenatal care All of the women had given prelacteal feeds to their babies

TABLE 94: Studies on perceived breast milk insufficiency

Method: Prospective studies

Authors	Date	Where published	Intervention assessed	Entry criteria	Number of women studied	Outcomes measured	Results
Hillervik-Lindquist C	1991	Acta Paediatr Scand Supplement 376: 6–27 *study also in: Acta Paediatr Scand* 80:297–303	No intervention As part of prospective follow-up women received home visits monthly and telephone contacts at least every two weeks, from 1 week to 6 months post-partum At each point of contact mothers were asked about their experience of, and attitude towards breastfeeding, and current breastfeeding behaviour Infant's breast milk intake was measured at 1 week, then monthly till 6 months. Infant weight was also recorded at these points, and also at 9, 12, 15 and 18 months	Mothers motivated to breastfeed, recruited from 'out-of-hospital unit' for women requiring 'light postnatal care' First five mothers admitted to the postnatal ward every week during Jan to Sept and half of Oct 1983 Infants were healthy, weighed >3kg at birth and breastfed exclusively on discharge	51 mother-infant pairs followed prospectively from 3 days to 18 months post-partum Mean length of total breastfeeding was 36 weeks (range 8–72); at 12 months 20% of the infants were still being breastfed	Incidence of 'lactation crises' Milk intake at time of transient lactation crisis Comparison of milk intake between groups Attitude to breastfeeding Infant growth Duration of breastfeeding	28 mothers out of 51 (55%) experienced 'transient lactation crisis' ('crisis' group), 23/51 (45%) did not – 'non-crisis' group Within crisis group, no difference in milk intake during 'crisis' compared with 'control' period 1 week later Milk intake in 'crisis' group consistently lower than in 'non-crisis' group throughout period of measurements; significantly lower at 3 and 5 months Women in 'crisis' group tended to give infant-related reasons for initiating breastfeeding, compared with mother-related reasons in 'non-crisis' group Infants in 'crisis' group were of significantly lower weight between 2–4 months of age and at 9 months Mother in 'crisis' group started weaning significantly earlier and also stopped breastfeeding earlier

TABLE 95: Improvement of defective lactation by using oral metoclopramide

Method: Randomised placebo-controlled trial

Authors	Date	Where published	Intervention assessed	Entry criteria	Number of women studied	Outcomes measured	Results		
							Normal lactating women (n=30)	MTC treated group (n=11)	Placebo and MTC treated group (n=10)
Guzman V Toscano G Canales ES Zarate A	1979	Acta Obstet Gynecol Scand 58: 53–55	Metoclopramide 10 mg twice daily for 4 weeks versus placebo In the control group of women that received the placebo, if they reported insufficient lactation in the 2nd week postpartum they were then given metoclopramide for the following 2 weeks	Women wishing to breastfeed with a previous history of poor lactation	21 Experimental group n=11 Control group n=10 30 normal lactating women were included as a comparison	Mean basal serum prolactin: 1st day postpartum Postpartum weeks: 2nd 3rd 4th	465.0±57.7 234.0±31.4 160.0±27.3 98.2±17.1	373.7±34.8 379.6±51.4 338.1±59.2 383.4±74.9	320.4±46.8 149.8±14.2 286.1±45.6 180.5±52.8

TABLE 96: Controlled trial of metoclopramide in the initiation of breast-feeding

Method: Randomised placebo-controlled trial

Authors	Date	Where published	Intervention assessed	Entry criteria	Number of women studied	Outcomes measured	Results
Lewis PJ Devenish C Kahn C	1980	Br J Clin Pharmac 9: 217–9	Metoclopramide 10 mg 3 times per day for 7 days post-operatively to caesarean section versus placebo Placebo group received lactose NB 2hr after a single dose to the mother the plasma and breast milk levels of metoclopramide were 68.5±29.6 and 125.7±41.7 ng/ml respectively, giving an estimated sub-therapeutic dose to the baby of 45 µg/kg	Women undergoing caesarean section deliveries	20 women 10 in treatment group 10 in placebo group	Success at establishing breastfeeding	No differences between treatment and placebo group in establishing breastfeeding, both groups were 100% successful at initiating breastfeeding and sustaining it till at least 6 weeks post-partum

TABLE 97: A dose response relation between improved lactation and metoclopramide

Method: Placebo-controlled cross-over study

Authors	Date	Where published	Intervention assessed	Entry criteria	Number of women studied	Outcomes measured	Results	
Kauppila A Kivinen S Ylikorkala O	1981	Lancet i: 1175–1177	1. Metoclopramide 5 mg x 3 t.d.s. for 14 days versus placebo for a further 14 days 2. Metoclopramide 10 mg x 3 t.d.s. for 14 days versus placebo for a further 14 days 3. Metoclopramide 15 mg x 3 t.d.s. for 14 days versus placebo for a further 14 days	Lactating women who reported insufficient milk yields, whose average yield was 30% or less than 165 ml/kg/day	37 Group 1: 10 Group 2: 13 Group 3: 14	**Serum Prolactin (ng/ml)**	Before	After therapy
						Group 1	68.9±53.2 Placebo	106.8±93.4 56.7±68.1
						Group 2	77.8±59.8 Placebo	175.8±112.4 34.2±23.1
						Group 3	44.9±33.7 Placebo	189.3±123.7 28.4±33.7
						Breastmilk/feed (ml)	Before	After therapy
						Group 1	92.4±42.5 Placebo	104.5±43.2 96.8±48.2
						Group 2	96.3±48.8 Placebo	138.8±51.7 106.8±35.6
						Group 3	80.3±63.1 Placebo	130.3±70.5 80.0±53.4
						Supplementary feeds per day (ml)	Before	After therapy
						Group 1	295±183 Placebo	358±230 428±249
						Group 2	294±193 Placebo	228±227 352±218
						Group 3	360±188 Placebo	313±226 424±261

TABLE 98: Metoclopramide increases prolactin release and milk secretion in puerperium without stimulating the secretion of thyrotropin and thyroid hormones

Method: Placebo-controlled cross-over study

Authors	Date	Where published	Intervention assessed	Entry criteria	Number of women studied	Outcomes measured	Results		
Kauppila A Kivinen S Ylikorkala O	1981	J Clinical Endocrinol & Metab 52: 436–9	Metoclopramide (MC) 10 mg x3 t.d.s. for 14 days versus placebo for a further 14 days *Maternal PRL levels responded to both TRH and MC administration, while maternal TSH levels only responded to TRH administration and not to MC*	Lactating women with insufficient lactation from within the first 14 days, up to 60 days post-partum and who had started giving supplementary feeds	17 14 of whom completed the protocol	Serum Prolactin (ng/ml) Breastmilk (ml/day) Supplementary feeds per day (ml)	**Before** 36.6±9.2 No effect on TSH, free T$_3$ or T$_4$ 432±55 348±61 NB *The decline in PRL and breastmilk per day after a one week pause in therapy relative to before therapy (and increase in supplementary formula), suggest a possible 'rebound effect' after withdrawal of metoclopramide. These changes were reversed by resuming therapy*	**After 3 wks therapy** 55.4±11.1 626±76 280±59	**After 1 wk pause** 19.5±7.6 390±73 526±68

TABLE 99: Metoclopramide and breastfeeding: efficacy and anterior pituitary responses of the mother and the child

Method: Randomised placebo-controlled double blind trial

Authors	Date	Where published	Intervention assessed	Entry criteria	Number of women studied	Outcomes measured	Results
Kauppila A Anunti P Kivinen S Kiovisto M Ruokonen A	1988	Eur J Obstet Gynecol Repro Biol 19: 19–22	Metoclopramide 10mg x3 daily starting at 4 to 20 weeks postpartum for 3 weeks versus placebo Impact of therapy on both maternal and infant serum levels of prolactin (PRL), thyroid stimulating hormone (TSH) and free thyroxine (fT₄)	Women who wanted to improve milk production	25 Control group n=14 Experimental group n=11	Mean basal serum prolactin: 1 week after therapy started 3 weeks after therapy started No effect on TSH or free thyroxine levels Estimated daily milk yield: 1 week after therapy started 2 weeks after therapy started 3 weeks after therapy started	Experimental group / Control group / Difference (units are μl) 315 ± 300 / 89.6 ± 60 / $+225$ 211 ± 131 / 68.5 ± 55 / $+142$ Approx. values from figure 1. n=8 / n=5 480mls / 480mls / 0 510mls / 500mls / –10 520mls / 420mls / +100 Maternal use of metoclopramide had no effect in infant serum levels of PRL, TSH or fT₄

TABLE 100: Metoclopramide and breast milk

Method: Randomised placebo-controlled double blind trial

Authors	Date	Where published	Intervention assessed	Entry criteria	Number of women studied	Outcomes measured	Results		
							Experimental group (units are ng/ml)	Control group	Difference
de Gezelle H Oogne W Ghiery M Dhont M	1983	Eur J Obstet Gynaecol Repro Biol 15: 31–36	Metoclopramide 10mg x3 daily from 1st–8th day postpartum versus Placebo	Normal mothers and babies	13 Control group n=6 Experimental group n=7	Mean basal serum prolactin: Day 3 Day 7 Day 21 Day 28 Estimated daily milk yield: Day 3 Day 5 Day 7 Mean	240.9±89.3 132.0±130.9 57.6±67.5 64.1±84.9 (units are ml) 50.7±14.6 82.9±11.1 81.4±17.7 75.4±13.2	225.0±148.1 120.4±97.2 47.8±48.6 70.5±81 41.7±24 52.5±10.8 59.2±18.6 51.1±10.9	+15.9 +12 +98 −6.4 +9 +30.4 +22.2 +24.3

TABLE 101: Augmentation of puerperal lactation by oral administration of sulpiride

Method: Random selection of nursing women

Authors	Date	Where published	Intervention assessed	Entry criteria	Number of women studied	Outcomes measured	Results		
							Experimental group (units are ng/ml)	Control group	Difference
Aono T Shioji T Aki T Hirota K Nomura A Kurachi K	1979	J Clin Endocrinol Metab 48: 478–482	Administration of sulpiride to enhance lactation 50mg x2 daily first 7 days postpartum versus No intervention	Tended to complain of lactational insufficiency	130 Control group = 64 Experimental group = 66	Mean basal serum prolactin (±SE): after delivery 2nd day 4th day (from fig 4) 6th day Mean daily milk yield (±SE) 1st day 3rd day 5th day	114.7±6.5 177.9±2.9 (156.0±10) 138.0±13.8 (units are ml/day) 26.7±7.9 247.1±15.4 483.1±24.0	105.8±6.9 122.1±8.9 (110.0±5 Est.) 93.8±8.1 12.5±4.6 188.1±18.2 370.9±24.5	+8.9 +55.8 +56 +44.2 +14.2 +59.0 +112.2

TABLE 102: Effect of sulpiride on poor puerperal lactation

Method: Randomised placebo-controlled trial

Authors	Date	Where published	Intervention assessed	Entry criteria	Number of women studied	Outcomes measured	Results		Difference
							Experimental group (units are ng/ml)	Control group	
Aono T Aki T Kolke K Kurachi K	1982	Amer J Obst Gynaecol 143(8): 927–32	Administration of sulpiride to enhance lactation. 50mg x2 daily from 3rd day postpartum for 4 days versus placebo Estimated daily milk yield sum of suckled milk and expressed milk	Women with total milk secretion not exceeding 50ml for first 3 days	96 Control group n=48 Experimental group n=48	Mean basal serum prolactin (±SE): after delivery 2nd day 3rd day 6th day	108.5±5.6 121.9±6.9 162.5±13.5 133.2±12.1	103.5±7.5 115.7±6.3 (108±6 est.) (102±8 est.)	+5.0 +6.2 +55 +31
						Estimated daily milk yield (±SE): (units ml/day) 1st day 3rd day 4th day 5th day	15.3±3.4 111.4±17.0 224.5±21.0 325.8±31.7	15.9±3.6 86.6±14.7 143.5±19.6 211.1±72.9	–0.9 +24.8 +81.0 +114.7
						Effect on discontinuation rate at 4 weeks: Primips.	4/20 (20%)	4/20 (20%)	No significant difference
						Multips.	3/20 (15%)	4/20 (20%)	Odds ratio 0.71

TABLE 103: Sulpiride improves inadequate lactation

Method: Randomised placebo-controlled double blind trial

Authors	Date	Where published	Intervention assessed	Entry criteria	Number of women studied	Outcomes measured	Results		
								Before	After
Ylikorkala O Kauppila A Kivinen S Viinikka L	1982	BMJ 285: 249–251	Sulpiride 50 mg x3 daily for 4 weeks versus Placebo	Women who reported having insufficient lactation in the first 4 months after delivery	26 Experimental group n=14 Control group n=12	Serum prolactin concentration	Experimental group: Increase from	49.0±3.6 mg/l	402.1±43.2 mg/l
							Control group: Decrease from	84.7±24.0 mg/l to	47.8 ± 8.6 mg/l
				Some women were excluded from the control group because of 'lack of effect from the treatment'		Milk yields	Experimental group: average increase of 212–265 ml		
							Control group: milk yields fell by 30–40 ml daily		

TABLE 104: Treatment of inadequate lactation with oral sulpiride and buccal oxytocin

Method: Double blind placebo controlled trial

Authors	Date	Where published	Intervention assessed	Entry criteria	Number of women studied	Outcomes measured	Results		
Ylikorkala O Kauppila A Kivinen S Viinikka L	1984	Obstet Gynaecol 63(1): 57–59	The first 24 women were treated in a double blind study of sulpiride versus placebo, plus buccal oxytocin Group 1: Oral sulpiride (150 mg) + buccal oxytocin (100 IU) versus placebo Larger doses of oxytocin were studied in an open trial with 12 women Group 2: Oral sulpiride (150 mg) + buccal oxytocin (300 IU, n=6 or 400 IU, n=6) Oral sulpiride or placebo taken 3 x day for 2 weeks; oxytocin given on day 6 and 14, 10 minutes prior to each feed, placebo on days 7 and 13	Women who in their initial 4 month period after delivery considered their lactation to be insufficient The breasts had to be anatomically healthy	36 Experimental Group 1: n=12 Experimental Group 2: n=12 Control group: n=12 *4 women left the trial because of lack of effect of treatment; 1 from sulpiride group, 3 from placebo*	Milk yield (±SE) on: Day 6/7 Day 13/14 Mean serum prolactin (±SE) at: 1 week 13–14 days	Experimental groups 1 and 2 (units are ml/day) 628±51 n=23 648±67 n=23 Experimental groups 1 and 2 (units are ml/day) 380±43 n=23 381±38 n=23 No differences in serum prolactin or milk yield were found in the comparison between buccal oxytocin (100–400 IU) and placebo	Control group 440±68 n=9 423±60 n=9 Control group 23±7 n=9 34±10 n=9	p<0.05 p<0.01 p<0.001 p<0.001

TABLE 105: Domperidone in defective and insufficient lactation

Method: Double blind randomised controlled trial

Authors	Date	Where published	Intervention assessed	Entry criteria	Number of women studied	Outcomes measured	Results		
							Experimental (units ng/ml)	Controls	Difference
Petraglia F de Leo V Sardelli S Pieroni ML D'Antona N Genazzani AR	1985	Eur J Obstet Gynecol Biol 19: 281–287	Effects of domperidone on prolactin levels and daily milk yields Group A: 10mg x 3 daily, 2nd to 5th postpartum day Group B: 10 postpartum days	Group A: Mulitps with a history of failure of lactogenesis in previous puerperium Group B: Primips affected by inadequate lactation 2 weeks after delivery	Group A: Controls n=7 Experimental n=8 Group B: Controls n=8 Experimental n=9	Mean basal serum prolactin Group A: Day 3 postpartum Day 5 postpartum Group B: 2nd treatment day Estimated daily milk yield Group B: 2nd treatment day 6th treatment day 10th treatment day	155 150 169±27 (units are ml/day) 347±36 636±59 672±44	98 70 84±17 335±30 440±27 398±45	+57 +80 +85 +12 +196 +275

TABLE 106: Domperidone: secretion in breastmilk and effect on puerperal prolactin levels

Method: Randomised placebo-controlled trial

Authors	Date	Where published	Intervention assessed	Entry criteria	Number of women studied	Outcomes measured	Results
Hofmeyr GJ van Iddekinge B Blott JA	1985	Br J Obstet Gynaecol, 92: 141–144	20mg Domperidone 1 dose only versus placebo	Mothers whose babies were temporarily unable to take breast-milk	10 Experimental group n=5 Control group n=5	Mean basal serum prolactin	Taken 2 hours after treatment Experimental group = 255 ng/ml Control group = 150 ng/ml Difference = +155 ng/ml

TABLE 107: Oral administration of TRH in puerperal women: effect on insufficient lactation, thyroid hormones and on the responses of TSH and prolactin to intravenous TRH

Method: Non-randomised prospective intervention study

Authors	Date	Where published	Intervention assessed	Entry criteria	Number of women studied	Outcomes measured	Results
Ylikorkala O Kivinen S Kauppila A	1980	Acta Endocrinol 93: 413–418	Intravenous thyrotrophin releasing hormone stimulation test Followed by: 20 mg thyrotrophin releasing hormone (TRH) twice daily for 2 weeks	Women with reported insufficient lactation, entering the study between weeks 3–10 postpartum	13	Mean basal prolactin levels	The mean prolactin levels decreased during the study Experimental Control 23.0±7.9 61.4±26.2 $p < 0.05$
						Mean thyrotrophin (TSH)	There was no change in TSH level
						T_3 & T_4 levels - T_3 - T_4	T_3 & T_4 levels elevated Experimental Control 2.17±0.14 1.8±0.1 $p < 0.01$ 131.6±7.9 96.6±5.8 $p < 0.01$
						Lactation response	No significant changes in milk production
							Side effects recorded included nausea and flushing

TABLE 108: Thyrotrophin-Releasing Hormone (TRH) – a lactation-promoting agent?

Method: Randomised double-blind placebo-controlled study

Authors	Date	Where published	Intervention assessed	Entry criteria	Number of women studied	Outcomes measured	Results	
Peters F Schulze-Tollert J Schuth W	1991	Brit J Obstet Gynaecol 98:880–885	TRH by nasal spray 1mg QDS between suckling episodes for 10 consecutive days, starting on 6th postpartum day	Women with output 50% less than "normal milk yield" (165g/kg/day*) on 5th postpartum day (*based on Editorial, BMJ 1954, 264–5, and test-weighing)	19 10 intervention 9 control (placebo spray)	Daily milk yield at (mean±SD): start of treatment 10th day Then: 5 days and 10 days after cessation of treatment 7 women treated for further 10 days	Experimental group (units are g/day) 142.0±33.9 253.0±105.3 p=0.014 239.0±123.3 254.4±121.9 no change 424.3±168.1	Control group 150.0±46.2 140.6±57.7 p=0.87 n.s. 146.7±52.2 161.1±60.3 no change
						Serum prolactin (normal for all pre-trial): start of treatment 10th day Serum thyroid hormones	Experimental group (units are microg/l) 117.4±45.2 173.3±55.5 p<0.001 No significant change in TSH, T4 and T3	Control group 137.2±69.5 82.0±37.7 p=0.016

TABLE 109a: The effect of oral administration of thyrotrophin-releasing hormone on lactation

Method: Double blind placebo-controlled trial

Authors	Date	Where published	Intervention assessed	Entry criteria	Number of women studied	Outcomes measured	Results		
							Experimental group	Control group	Difference
Zarate A Villalobos H Canales E Soria J Arcovedo F MacGregor C	1976	J Clin Endocrinol Metab 43: 301–305	60mg of thyrotrophin-releasing hormone versus placebo The drug or the placebo was given from 2 days postpartum until 4 weeks postpartum	Healthy women who had previously breastfed successfully	16 Experimental group n=8 Control group n=8	Mean basal serum prolactin measured on: Day 7 postpartum Day 14 postpartum Day 21 postpartum Day 28 postpartum	 550ng/ml 540ng/ml 230ng/ml 170ng/ml	 155ng/ml 120ng/ml 100ng/ml 80ng/ml	 +395 +420 +130 +90

TABLE 109b: The effect of oral administration of thyrotrophin-releasing hormone on lactation

Method: Double blind placebo-controlled trial – Conjoint study

Authors	Date	Where published	Intervention assessed	Entry criteria	Number of women studied	Outcomes measured	Results
Zarate A Villalobos H Canales E Soria J Arcovedo F MacGregor C	1976	J Clin Endocrinol Metab 43: 301–305	Thyrotrophin-releasing hormone versus placebo	Women with inadequate lactation	8 Experimental group n=4 Control group n=4	Mean basal serum prolactin Milk yield	There was no increase in basal serum prolactin in the experimental group There was no increase in milk yield in the experimental group

TABLE 110: Growth hormone stimulates galactopoiesis in healthy lactating women

Method: Double blind randomised placebo-controlled trial

Authors	Date	Where published	Intervention assessed	Entry criteria	Number of women studied	Outcomes measured	Results
Milsom SR Breier BH Gallaher BW Cox VA Gunn AJ Gluckman PD	1992	Acta Endocrinologica 127: 337–343	Human growth hormone 0.1 IU/Kg versus placebo Administered by injection pen at 09.00 on days 3 to 9 of study	Healthy breastfeeding women; 18–40 years; no known contra-indications to growth hormone therapy; on no medication Infants: Term, healthy with no feeding difficulties; between 8–18 weeks postpartum	16	Mean breastmilk volumes Milk composition Milk and plasma growth hormone levels	On study day 1 Experimental group n=8 mean vol = 835 mls standard deviation = 64 mls Control group n=8 mean vol = 855 mls standard deviation = 65 mls On study day 10 Experimental group n=8 mean vol = 992 mls standard deviation = 79 mls Control group n=8 mean vol = 955 mls standard deviation = 71 mls No significant difference in milk composition between groups All women in the experimental group showed an increase in human growth hormone but the values remained within the values observed in the control group

TABLE 111: A herbal drug that stimulates lactation

Method: Non-randomised, uncontrolled study

Authors	Date	Where published	Intervention assessed	Entry criteria	Number of women studied	Outcomes measured	Results
Gokhale M	1965	Indian Practitioner 18(9): 665–70	Given herbal drug Leptaden (Alarsen) (Normal dose 2 tabs t.d.s.)	Breastfeeding women in hospital, giving a history of lactation failure	25	Lactation following administration of Leptaden (only the results from 11 of the cases)	Lactation appears to have been increased following administration of the drug. However most were pronounced to have lactation failure on 3rd, or 4th day, and the quantity of milk expressed was measured on about day 3–4 of treatment

TABLE 112: Randomized controlled trial of *Asparagus racemosus* (Shatavari) as a lactogogue in lactational inadequacy

Method: A randomised placebo controlled trial

Authors	Date	Where published	Intervention assessed	Entry criteria	Number of women studied	Outcomes measured	Results
Sharma S Ramji S Kumari S Bapna JS	1996	Indian Pediatrics 3: 675–677	Women with insufficient milk were randomised to receive either: 1. Galactogogue 2 tsf. twice daily for 4 weeks or 2. A placebo 2 tsf. twice daily for 4 weeks Each 100 g of galactogogue contained Shatavari 15.0 g, as the active principle along with other herbal ingredients.	Women who had delivered term healthy infants. Between 14–90 days postpartum Reported having insufficient milk All mothers with the diagnosis of 'lactational inadequacy' were encouraged to breastfeed exclusively, taught correct positioning and advised on adequate rest and nutrition Following 1 week of exclusive breastfeeding mothers whose infants had failed to gain >15 g/day were included in the study	64 Group 1: 32 Group 2: 32 11 (17.2.%) failed to complete the trial	1. Maternal PRL levels (ng/ml) 2. Infant weight gain velocity (g/d) 3. Volume of supplemental milk	There was no increase in maternal PRL levels There was a significant increase in infant weight gain and a decrease in amounts of supplements given in both groups. This was probably a result of improved breastfeeding technique The study concluded that *Asparagus racemosus* had no lactogogic effect

TABLE 113: Incidence of Hyperbilirubinaemia in breast vs formula-fed infants

Method: Retrospective study

Authors	Date	Where published	Method	Entry criteria	Number of women studied	Outcomes measured	Results
Adams JA Hey DJ Hall RT	1985	Clinical Pediatrics 24(2): 69–73	A number of variables were examined from the case notes, to see if it possible to predict babies that might develop hyperbilirubinaemia Variables included: - Method of delivery - Any bruising or minor birth injuries - Birth weight - Method of feeding	Gestational age >38 weeks Born in 1980 at the study hospital Exclusions: ABO incompatibility with positive direct Coombs test No follow-up visit within 4 weeks	233 101 breastfed 117 formula fed 15 babies with cephalo-haematoma were excluded from analysis	Incidence of hyperbilirubinaemia in the 1st week of life >12 mg/dl >15 mg/dl	Significantly more breastfed babies (p<0.02) Significantly more breastfed babies (p<0.002) All breastfed infants in the study received water supplementation after feeding, and many had also received 2–3 formula feedings. Most also received less than 8 feeds in 24 hours because of perceived difficulties in carrying out 'breastfeed on demand' instructions

TABLE 114: Frequency of breast-feeding and serum bilirubin concentration

Method: Descriptive study

Authors	Date	Where published	Intervention assessed	Entry criteria	Number of women studied	Outcomes measured	Results
de Carvalho M Klaus MH Merkatz RB	1982	Am J Dis Child 136: 737–738	All mothers were encouraged to feed their babies whenever they thought they were hungry The mother kept a feed chart for 3 days Supplements were not given following breastfeeds For data analysis the babies were divided into two groups: Group 1: Mean frequency of feeding was >8 feeds in 24 hours Group 2: Mean frequency of feeding was <8 feeds in 24 hours	Primiparous, uncomplicated pregnancy and delivery Planned to breastfeed The babies were normal at birth Birth weight between 3000–4000 g Breastfed within 1 hour following delivery	55 mother and baby pairs	Frequency of feeding in 24 hours Serum bilirubin Weight loss	Group 1: < 8 feeds in 24 hours = 6.8 ± 0.8 Group 2: > 8 feeds in 24 hours = 10.1 ± 1.6 Group 1: < 8 feeds in 24 hours = 9.3 mg/dL ± 3.5 mg/dL Group 2: > 8 feeds in 24 hours = 6.6 mg/dL ± 4.0 mg/dL Group 1: < 8 feeds in 24 hours = 219g ± 86g Group 2: > 8 feeds in 24 hrs = 216g ± 59g

TABLE 115: Hospital routines in infants with hyperbilirubinemia influence the duration of breastfeeding

Method: Non-randomised prospective study

Authors	Date	Where published	Intervention assessed	Entry criteria	Number of women studied	Outcomes measured	Results
Elander G Lindberg T	1986	Acta Paediatr Scand 75: 708–712	Infants who were receiving phototherapy were divided into two groups: 1. Separated group, these babies were transferred to the children's ward and their mothers remained on postnatal ward, they were free to visit and care for their babies. 2. Non-separated group, these mothers and babies stayed together in a single room, they were taught how to care for their babies by one of the investigators. 3. Control group, these mothers cared for their babies in the single room for 24 hours	Healthy babies between the ages of 37–41 weeks gestation who developed jaundice were included over 15 month recruiting period	Group 1 = 15 Group 2 = 14 Control group = 55	Urine cortisol levels in the mothers Breastfeeding duration	No significant difference was found in the urine cortisol between the groups The results given, showed a p<0.05 between groups 1 and 2, this demonstrated that more of the mothers were still breastfeeding at 12 weeks in the group that had not been separated for the period of treatment

TABLE 116: Breastfeeding patterns: Comparing the effects on infant behavior and maternal satisfaction of using one or two breasts

Method: Randomised controlled trial

Authors	Date	Where published	Intervention assessed	Entry criteria	Number of women studied	Outcomes measured	Results
Righard L Flodmark C-E Lothe L Jakobsson I	1993	Birth 20(4): 182–5	Mothers assigned in hospital to either a one or a two breast per feed pattern	Healthy mothers, 3–4 days after delivery. All breastfeeding exclusively in hospital, and using two breasts per feed. 103 women approached	80 consenting mothers, randomly allocated to either the one breast/feed group (n=44), or the two breast/feed group (n=36)	Compliance	Poor compliance in one-breast per feed (16/33) compared with two-breast per feed group (26/27) (p<0.001)
						Periods of sleep, restlessness, and crying	No significant differences in sleep, restlessness, and crying
					Only 60 women were breastfeeding exclusively at 1 month follow-up (33:27)	Cases of colic	1 in one-breast group 4 in two-breast group (not significant)
						Mother's satisfaction, mood and confidence at 1 month post-partum	No significant differences
					'Approved records' were completed by 36 (13:23), i.e. drop-out rates 71% and 25%	Frequency of feeds, wet nappies and loose stools	Comparable between groups

TABLE 117: Breastfeeding in infants with Down's syndrome

Method: Survey

Authors	Date	Where published	Intervention assessed	Entry criteria	Number of women studied	Outcomes measured	Results
Aumonier ME Cunningham CC	1983	Child: Care, Health and Development 9: 247–255	Parents informally interviewed at home as part of an early intervention programme by health visitors	Babies born in Greater Manchester, 1.2.76–28.2.78 with chromosomally-confirmed Down's Syndrome; and their mothers Fostered babies included (n=7) Babies in institutional care excluded	61 babies of which 26 were breastfed	Antenatal wish to breastfeed Started to breastfeed Breastfed >1 month Poor sucking ability Support from hospital staff to breastfeed	54% (n=29) 48% (n=26) 16/29 Associated with severe cardiac anomalies 70% of mothers – yes 30% of mothers – no Support helped mothers of babies slow to suck. Knowledge that they are likely to succeed might help more mothers start to feed Down's syndrome babies

TABLE 118: Early repair and breastfeeding for infants with cleft lip
1. Retrospective-cleft lip repairs 2. Choice to breastfeed soon after cleft lip surgery

Method: Case series

Authors	Date	Where published	Intervention assessed	Entry criteria	Number of women studied	Outcomes measured	Results
Weatherly-White RCA Knehn DP Mirrett P Gilman JI Weatherly-White CC	1987	Plastic and Reconstructive Surgery 79(6): 879–885	1. Timing of surgery to correct cleft lip* 2. All mothers of babies having surgery for cleft lip* offered opportunity of breastfeeding after repair *Unclear when cleft lip only, or cleft lip and palate is meant	1. 100 conservative cleft lip* repairs by same surgeon 1970–1978 2. Series of 60 babies from 1983	100 38 began to breastfeed within hours of surgery 16 continued for 6 weeks or more The rest started cups/ naso-gastric feeding and went on to bottle	1. Operative morbidity and mortality 2. Surgical and post-operative complications Birthweight, weight at operation and at 3 months Duration of hospital stay	Significantly fewer complications at 1 week old or less No difference when surgery was at 1–3 weeks or more than 3 weeks 15 of 16 successful breastfeeding babies had cleft lip only The only complication was partial dehiscence in a cup-feeding baby The cupfeeding babies gained less weight than breast or bottle feeding babies The breastfeeding babies stayed in hospital less time

TABLE 119: Breastfeeding or spoon feeding after cleft lip repair

Method: A prospective randomised study

Authors	Date	Where published	Intervention assessed	Entry criteria	Number of women studied	Outcomes measured	Results		
Darzi M A Chowdri N A Bhat A N	1996	British Journal of Plastic Surgery 49:24–26	Infants with cleft lip were studied over a 2 year period All lips were repaired under general anaesthetic by the same surgeon Following repair mothers and infants were randomly allocated to either: 1. Breastfeed or 2. Spoon feed	All infants with cleft lip alone between the age of 3–6 months Excluded were infants with associated cleft palate and more than 6 months	40	Weight at time of surgery Weight 3 weeks after surgery Weight 6 weeks after surgery Duration of hospital stay Rate of dehiscence	Group Breast Spoon Breast Spoon Breast Spoon Group Breast Spoon There was only one wound dehiscence in the 40 infants, in the spoon group	Mean wt in kg 5.02±0.57 5.15±0.48 5.85±0.64 5.55±0.53 6.35±0.48 5.88±0.37 Mean hospital stay (days) 5.80±0.88 6.00±1.12	p value >0.20 >0.10 <0.01

TABLE 120: Neonatal frenotomy may be necessary to correct breastfeeding problems

Method: Case studies

Authors	Date	Where published	Intervention assessed	Entry criteria	Number of women studied	Outcomes measured	Results
Marmet C Shell E Marmet R	1990	J Hum Lact 6(3): 117–121	Analysis of tight frenulum cases in 1988	Short frenulum on visual assessments Seen at the Lactation Institute for Breastfeeding Problems	13 babies	10 babies were recommended for frenotomy Breastfeeding following frenotomy Breastfeeding when frenotomy was recommended but not performed	6 breastfeeding with no problem 1 unresponsive: severe retardation was suspected 3 cases: 1. Breastfeeding, but mother had milk supply problems and sore nipples 2. Breast and bottle feeding 3. Stopped breastfeeding

TABLE 121: The importance of the identification of ankyloglossia (short lingual frenulum) as a cause of breastfeeding problems

Method: 2 case histories

Authors	Date	Where published	Results
Notestine GE	1990	J Hum Lact 6(3): 113–115	Two case studies were discussed Ankyloglossia identified Nipple pain and trauma relieved. Follow-up not reported (Both mothers breastfed twice previously) Very good photographs and descriptions More references on tongue-tie Good points about educating primagravidae "There may be no problem . . . if mother's breast is small, elastic and has reservoirs close to the nipple"